Beyond 60™
Massage for Mature Adults

Mary L. Duval

Beyond 60™
Massage for Mature Adults
Mary L. Duval

© Mary L. Duval 2015

Dedication

My thanks to everyone who made this book possible:

My instructors from the Lauterstein-Conway Massage School who gave me the skills necessary to perform the massage that I love.

My clients for allowing me to work with them and gain the understanding of how to work with mature adults.

My mother for being one of my first mature adult clients.

My editor for helping to bring this book to completion.

Table of Contents

Introduction

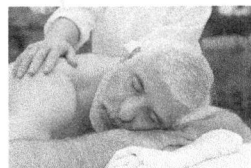 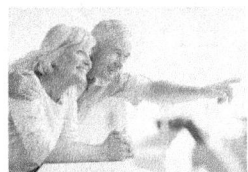 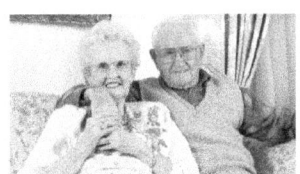

When I went to massage school I was looking for a career change. I had spent the majority of 18 years working in an office, most of that time working in the computer industry doing technical writing. While I had learned a lot and had some fun along the way, I was tired of the grind of writing manuals and working for customers who were always on to the next crisis as soon as their latest release was delivered.

I had spent a couple years thinking about what I wanted to do and researching possibilities. I knew I wasn't looking to go back to college. I needed something that was more enjoyable and fulfilling while also paying the bills. I had spent several years trying other things (home party sales, real estate, running a cookie business, multilevel marketing, country music website, etc.) and I found that I could either enjoy what I did or make money, but having both was difficult.

Because I had received massage for almost 20 years, I knew the relaxation and therapeutic results that could be achieved. I also knew that, overall, it would be a job where people would look forward to and appreciate the work that I did.

When I started massage school, I still wasn't 100% sure it was what I wanted to do. I had had enough false starts to know that massage might not be my answer. However, after just a couple weeks in class I was hooked!

It was in massage school that I first had an inkling about working with mature adults. I was thinking about my career longevity and I had thought that if I built a solid client base who were in their 40s or 50s at that point, I might be able to have clients for a long time, long into their aging process. Also during my training, I ended up working with a lot of folks who were in their 60s and 70s as part of my outside massage experience. I started realizing then that mature adults (seniors) were not just frail old people who only needed light massage.

As my training was coming to an end, I had to decide what path my life would take next. My original thoughts were to work for someone else for a period of time while trying to build my personal business in my spare time. My ultimate goal was always to build my own business. All my different work adventures in the past had taught me that I loved running my own business. But, I knew building a business would take time and I needed money coming in sooner rather than later.

Then, just as I was about to graduate, I found someone who was looking to sell her outcall business in a 55-and-older community not too far from where I lived. Basically, I had the opportunity to walk out of massage school and into my own business! I began to believe that perhaps I was finally on the right track.

I explored the details of the business and realized that it was a great opportunity. I made a deal and had the beginnings of my business by the time I graduated from massage school. I was on my way!

Mature adults are now my bread and butter. Most of my clients are in their 60s and 70s, with several in their 80s, and even one or two in their 90s! With the baby boomers aging, this group is growing. Seven to ten thousand people turn 60 each day here in the United States and they're looking for massage!

Knowing that mature adults are a growing population, I realized that this was an opportunity for growth. I knew I would eventually hit the maximum number of clients I could work on in a week. After about a year and a half of working as a massage therapist, I decided that I should start a business with massage therapists working for me who also focus on working with mature adults. That way, we could help even more mature adults! This business is still growing and I don't see it slowing down any time soon.

I have found that selecting mature adults for my clientele is one of the best decisions I ever made in my life. I have finally found that mix of doing a job that I like while making money (an enviable position to be sure)! My clients are happy to see me when I arrive and even happier when I leave. I feel good to be able to help them and I love the fact that I have therapists who are helping even more people. Our mature adult clients appreciate the work we do and I can tell you that I will never find a more grateful group of people to work with.

I decided to write this book because I believe the massage industry is missing information on working with mature adults. There is a wealth of information on working with healthy, young and middle-age clients. There is also a lot of information about working with geriatric clients (The Daybreak Institute is the leader in this area). But, we are missing information on mature adults – those who are past middle-age, but not yet geriatric. For the most part, mature adults seem to get mixed in with geriatric and can sometimes be referred to as "robust geriatric." In my mind, that's kind of like trying to stick a square peg in a round hole.

Most mature adults are not geriatric clients. They are active and fairly healthy. I define mature adults as those who are 60 years or older. So, some mature adults could require a geriatric massage, depending on their health and body condition, but most mature adults fall somewhere between middle-age and geriatric. They may have a few physical issues or aches and pains, but they're still very active and generally healthy. What we need to be able to do as massage therapists is evaluate the client before us and understand how to work with that client with his or her individual body condition. That is what this book is about.

I hope this book will give you the confidence to work with mature adults and to understand how massage for this group differs from geriatric massage and how best to serve this population. People in their 60s, 70s, 80s, and even 90s are still vital human beings and we owe it to them to serve them in the best possible manner.

Introduction

Chapter 1 – What is a Mature Adult?

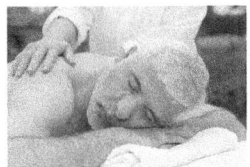 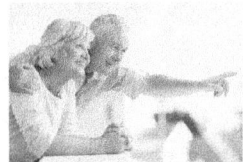 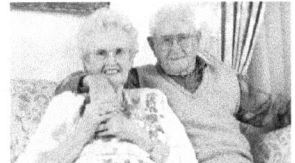

Introduction

Today, more people are living longer and are staying healthier in the process. While it is not new for people to live into their 70s, 80s, and 90s, there are many factors that have made it possible for more of them to live longer. The infant mortality rate has declined and advances have been made in medicine. Crime is down. Workplace safety has improved. All these things have made it possible for people to live longer. This means that we have larger numbers of older people in our communities and in our lives than we have had in the past.

This chapter will explore the definition of mature adults and examine what their lives are like.

Terminology

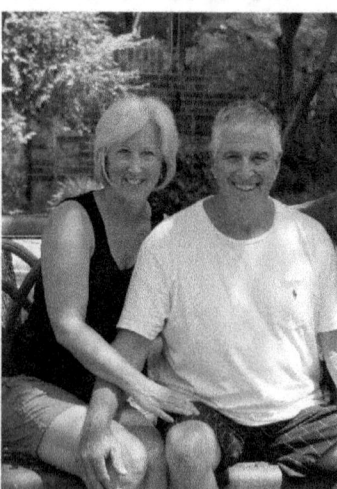

Senior?

Elder?

Geriatric?

Elderly?

Terminology!

Over the years we have used several terms to describe the older folks in our lives. As with many words in our language, how those terms are used and how they are received has changed over time.

In the massage industry, we use geriatric massage to describe massage that is performed on anyone who is 65 or older. When I started working with senior citizens, I told people that I did senior massage. From the beginning, I never saw myself as doing much geriatric massage. When I had used the term "senior" with other massage therapists or students, though, they immediately assumed I was working with frail, old people and doing geriatric massage. At first, I thought this was just a terminology problem and that I could explain away these misconceptions. However, I eventually realized this might not be a problem I could correct.

I had an enlightening conversation with another therapist one day. She said she wasn't interested in working with seniors because they usually needed a really light massage, needed a lot of work to get them into a comfortable position on the massage table, and they usually couldn't afford to get much massage. This does not describe the majority of the clients I work with!

When I explained to this therapist that my seniors were still very active, in good health, and financially comfortable, she admitted that she would be interested in working with my type of seniors! So, there was a disconnect between how I thought of seniors and how others thought of them.

The term "geriatric" relates more to "a branch of medicine that deals with the problems and diseases of old age and aging people or an aged person" (miriamwebster.com). The last part of that definition ("an aged person") implies people who are well beyond their prime and probably have a lot of health or physical issues. However, there is no specific age or description that tells you when a person is geriatric — you just have to "know" it.

The problem with the term "geriatric" is that while we can use the term to talk about a branch of medicine, or even a specific type of massage, we can NEVER call a person "geriatric." According to the online Oxford Dictionaries, "When used outside such contexts, it typically carries overtones of being worn out and decrepit and can therefore be offensive if used with reference to people." So, avoid this term when talking to and about your older clients!

Elderly is another term that has negative connotations. The term is fairly generic and is used to discuss people who are in the later stages of life or who are rather old. This term doesn't describe body condition or a specific age, but many times it conveys a feeling of someone who is feeble or not in good health. Even when you are talking about a person who is very old and frail, referring to them as elderly can raise some hackles!

So, what about "senior"? The term "senior citizen" is an official term used by governments to indicate when a person is eligible for retirement benefits. In this instance it means that a person is 65 (in the United States, 60 in other countries) years of age or older and nothing more. There is no inherent description of the health or energy level of the person. It's a numerical age only. However, even this term has begun to take on a negative connotation among seniors themselves (usually younger seniors)!

Another term that is used a lot is "elder." This term is a bit different because it is meant to honor the person being referred to. It is a word of respect, but, again, when is someone an "elder"? Also, not everyone really wants to be referred to as an elder, because it can conjure up the image of a wrinkled old person.

In our society, we tend to use the terms "senior," "elderly," and "geriatric" interchangeably when describing older adults. Sometimes these terms are used as a way to dismiss an older person. That's not always the case, but we should use these terms carefully.

A problem I see in the massage community is that we tend to talk about all senior massage as geriatric massage. But is that really fair? Geriatric massage makes it sound like you are working on really old people in poor health. I work on many people in their 60s and 70s and even some in their 80s whom I would not classify as geriatric. In my opinion, geriatric is a subset of senior massage, not the other way around.

I often run across articles with a title mentioning senior massage and I get excited to read something about seniors. Unfortunately, usually by the second or third paragraph it is clear that the article is addressing geriatric clients, not seniors. Because most of my clients are seniors and NOT geriatric, this disappoints me. I want to know more about my clients!

What I am seeing these days is that people don't think of themselves as old (or even getting older) and they don't want to be reminded that they are getting older. Thanks to better health, many older folks are still extremely active and aren't in much worse condition than someone in their 40s or 50s.

However, no matter how someone may feel about getting older, the truth is that people do age. And as they age, they can run into more illnesses, conditions, and diseases that younger people don't have. Many of those conditions may be manageable and no longer life threatening, but age-related problems do still happen.

After a lot of thought and search for alternative terms to use, I finally settled on "mature adult" to describe the clients I work with and most people agree this is a good term. For me, a mature adult is someone who is 60 years of age or older. This creates a big range in health conditions from hale and hearty to frail. The key to addressing this large population is knowing how to evaluate these clients (discussed in Chapter 5) and then providing the massage that meets their needs and the requirements of their body.

In this book, I focus mostly on healthier mature adults. I do briefly mention geriatric massage issues from time to time because you may run into geriatric clients when working with mature adults, but this is not an exhaustive discussion of geriatric massage. If you want to work with truly geriatric clients (defined in Chapter 2) then you will want to connect with the Daybreak Institute and get training from them. They pioneered geriatric massage and have the knowledge and techniques that will allow you to succeed with this population.

This book focuses on mature adults and the conditions you might encounter, but which will not incapacitate your clients. For example, a pacemaker won't stop you from doing a full 60 or 90 minute massage, but you may have to make adjustments to make your client comfortable on the table. Or, a knee replacement may slow your client down, but they won't be incapacitated for good and you can help with their recovery. A client with severe Parkinson's, though, is a geriatric massage client.

The Baby Boomers

The baby boomers are here! A baby boomer is someone who was born after World War II, from 1946 to 1964. During this time there was a large increase in the birth rate, creating a LOT of baby boomers. Thanks to this group, the number of people who are 65 is growing at a tremendous rate. As of 2011, 7,000 to 10,000 people turn 65 every day in the United States! This will continue until December 31st, 2030, when the last baby boomer will turn 65.

What this means is that we will have a LOT of mature adults who will need massage for many years to come. Of course, there will always be mature adults in need of massage, but right now we have a big influx of these clients and they will want massage!

Knowing how to work with these clients will be key to the success of your massage practice. Even if you don't want to focus solely on this group, you will be seeing more of them walking through your door.

Health Issues

As we age, the body and mind can start to deteriorate. The rate of this deterioration is specific to each individual. Some people stay and look healthy for a long time, prompting friends and strangers to comment on how young they look and act and question if they are really the age they are (many of my clients fall into this category). On the other hand, there are many people whose health fades faster and they can look and act a lot older than they are.

What causes this difference in how people age? There are a lot of factors that influence how we age and I'm sure there are a lot of things we still don't know about. But there are several things we DO know about that affect aging. These include:

- injuries when we were young
- illnesses and conditions when we were young
- lifelong nutrition and health care throughout our lives
- bad habits throughout life
- genetics

Injuries

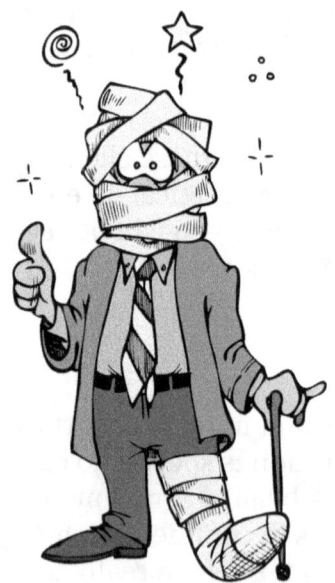

Ouch!

When we're young, we tend to bounce back quickly if we fall or hurt ourselves. It may be painful for a little while, but soon we're back out on the playground having a good time. If we break a bone, we heal and then move on, most of the time, forgetting that it even happened. However, those injuries stay with us. They may disappear from our consciousness for many years, but as we get older, those old injuries can make themselves known again.

Arthritis and aches and pains can be the result of a long-ago injury. Many times I've asked clients about problem areas and they cannot tell me how an injury happened because it occurred so long ago. Sometimes though, they will remember what happened and tell me the tale (usually a youthful indiscretion).

The difficult part about long-ago injuries is that the older they are, the less we can usually do for them. If an injury is 40, 50, or 60 years old, the chances of fixing it are slim. Usually, at this point all you can do is make your client feel better, at least temporarily.

And as we get older, it takes longer to recover when we get sick or injured. You will find that your mature adult clients will be more concerned about preventing new injuries, because they know it is harder to recover at their age. For example, they may have concerns about getting on and off your table or turning over because they are afraid of falling.

Illnesses/Conditions

While we've done a good job of getting rid of many diseases over the years (such as polio), many of our current mature adults are experiencing the results of these long ago illnesses and conditions.

Untreated scoliosis is a problem I've run across several times in my practice. In the past, we didn't have detection methods or treatments for the condition so nothing was done to correct the problem. Even now, some problems can be overlooked and won't be treated early.

I've had several clients who have had untreated scoliosis and are in their 80s. At this point, the spinal problems just compound the aging process and the client is usually in constant pain. Massage can make them feel better for a day or two, but the underlying problem is not fixed and can't be at this point. As a result, we have to do what we can, knowing we can't "fix" our clients.

Post-Polio Syndrome (PPS) affects polio survivors years after recovery from polio. Although polio has been eradicated in the United States and efforts to eradicate it from the rest of the world is progressing, you may still run into clients with PPS (see Chapter 6 for more information).

I'm sure that there are many other conditions which I have not yet run across that you might see. What's important to remember when you run into these issues is to do your best to make you client feel comfortable during the session and help them to the best of your ability.

Lifelong Nutrition and Health Care

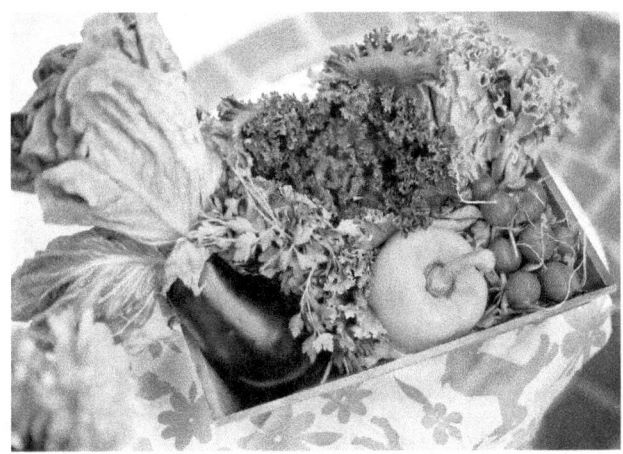

Healthy Eating

How we eat and the quality of health care we receive throughout our lives can greatly influence how we age.

If we don't get the proper nutrition in any stage in life, our bodies will not be able to function properly. Whether this happens when we are younger or older, poor nutrition can lead to illness and premature aging.

If we eat an unhealthy diet at a young age, but get better nutrition as we get older, we can greatly improve our health. But if we start eating a less healthy diet at an older age, when our bodies are less able to function without good nutrition, we could be in trouble.

As with proper nutrition, health care is very important when we are younger as well as when we get older. If we don't get proper preventative health care or don't take care of illnesses or conditions as soon as possible, problems can develop or get worse. When we don't get proper health care we are more susceptible to other illnesses or problems. Mature adults can be greatly affected by either past poor health care or current lapses in health care. Whether someone refuses to take proper care of themselves or a health care provider is not being as proactive as they should be, these issues can cause problems for an aging person. As with most things, the sooner a problem is rectified the better off people will be.

Bad Habits

If a person drinks to excess regularly throughout his or her life and/or is a heavy smoker, this will have a great impact on how that person ages. We can develop bad habits at any stage in life. If our poor health habits begin when we're young, we might be able to correct any damage from that habit if we change it soon enough. Bad habits that we develop as we get older, though, may be harder to get rid of and we may not recover as quickly from them.

People who have been sedentary a good portion of their lives may not have good mobility as they get older. Joints that are accustomed to being in a certain position my get stuck, and trying to unstick them and get them to move more freely will be a tough and, possibly, very painful process that clients may not want to go through.

Someone who is overweight, especially at an older age, may have mobility issues and may have trouble getting around. As we age, it's harder to lose weight so it can be very difficult for mature adults who are overweight.

Genetics

Genetics is kind of like a trump card in many ways. For those who have "good genes" it almost doesn't matter what they do in life. They can eat too much, drink too much, or smoke, but they will live a long life without many major problems. But, for those who have "bad genes" it almost doesn't matter how well they take care of themselves. They can eat healthy, exercise, never touch alcohol or smoke, but they will die early or have more than their share of health problems.

How long people live also seems to be primarily a function of genetics. We have all known families that seem to have longevity in their bloodlines with most of the family members living well into their 90s. Then there are other families that don't seem to make it much past the 70s or early 80s.

While geneticists keep working on the secrets of our genes, at this point there's not much we can do to fight the cards our genes deal us.

Staying Healthy Longer

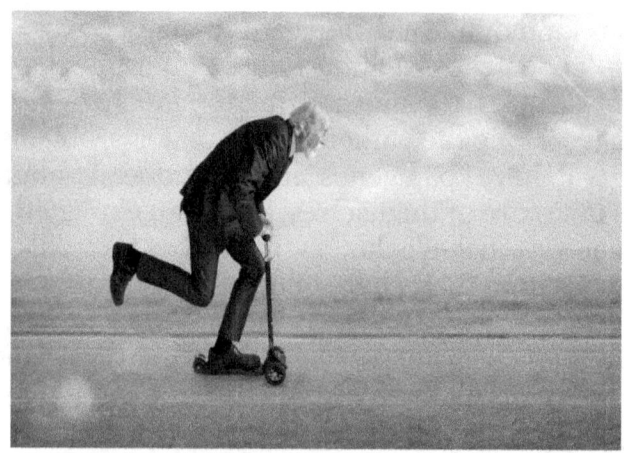

Fun is Ageless!

The good news today is that people are staying healthy longer. Thanks to better information and nutrition and increased and improved health care as well as an interest in alternative methods of staying healthy, many people are living longer and healthier lives.

There was a time in the US when making it to 70, 80, and 90 was considered a great achievement. As discussed earlier in this book, though, it is much more common for people to survive that long today.

Today, 60 is quite often a LONG way away from end of life. Many people are still working or volunteering at this age. They are active, participating in sports, traveling, getting together with friends, and hosting parties. Many don't look their age (or maybe we need to adjust what a 70 year old looks like!). It's not unusual to have people still active and healthy well into their 70s, 80s, and even 90s!

People are also realizing that the more they take care of themselves, the better they'll feel throughout their lives. They also know that massage and other alternative treatments will aid them in having a long and healthy life.

In Need of Massage

Because people are living longer they want to make sure they feel and move as well as they can. Many have discovered that taking medications to alleviate aches and pains is not the best way to handle these issues. They're learning that massage is a great way to relieve aches and pains and improve their range of motion and flexibility without pills or surgery. When they feel and move well they can enjoy their lives more.

Many people are also discovering that massage is an alternative treatment to common problems. Conditions such as carpal tunnel and sciatica can often be corrected or relieved without surgery. Those who suffer with these problems are now turning to massage before trying more invasive procedures.

As we age and physiological issues take hold, massage can be the perfect way to manage many of the effects of aging, and many mature adults are embracing this alternative treatment.

Place in Life

When people reach 60, they have usually done a lot in their lives. They have probably raised a family, traveled, and worked most of their lives. They have had struggles and laughs. They may be happy with their life as they look back on it or they may have regrets, or a little of both. They may have lots of friends and family around them or they may be lonely.

Where a person find themselves in the later years of life can have a great effect on their outlook on life and how well they take care of themselves. Massage can help them feel better if they are depressed (see Chapter 6 for details on depression).

When clients feel and move better, they may feel better about their lives. When someone is in a lot of constant pain, it can be hard for that person to be happy with their life. But massage can make that person feel better and give them the feeling that things may not be as bad as they thought.

If a person is happy with where they are in life, even proud they've made it as far as they have, massage will enhance these feelings. They will then spread their good mood to others.

For clients who are lonely, a visit from a massage therapist can really help. They have a visitor for a while who will give them the caring touch they are missing.

Although massage therapists are not life coaches, psychiatrists, or counselors, the work we do with massage can have great psychological benefits for our mature adult clients. When we help people feel better, their outlook on life improves from wherever they start.

Don't Generalize About Older People

I've often heard people say, "Oh, I love seniors. They're so sweet!" Well, some of them really are. And others, not so much. I always tell people that if someone was a pain to deal with when they were younger, they will be a pain to deal with when they're older. Yes, some people can and do change, but just because someone is 60 or older, it doesn't mean they're all of a sudden a sweet, nice person.

We also often hear about how older people are lonely and depressed. While this is certainly true for some mature adults, there are many who are having the time of their lives with friends and family around them. And then there are the people in between. They may not be totally happy, but over all, they're doing all right.

Mature adults are like any other clients we have. They are all individuals. We cannot say that all people over 60 are sweet. Or all people over 60 are mean. Nor can say all people over 60 are rich, or poor, or happy, or depressed. So we can't generalize about personality, outlook on life, or socioeconomic status.

We can make some general statements about the physical effects of aging, but not all age-related conditions will affect all mature adults. There is, however, more of a chance that we will see clients with some age-related conditions.

So, we need to treat each mature adult as the individual they are and design our massage sessions for that specific client.

Chapter 2 – What is Massage for Mature Adults?

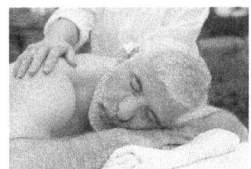 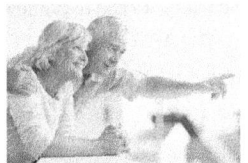 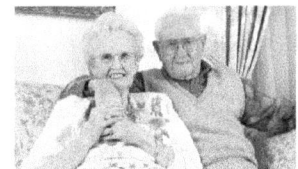

As described previously, a mature adult is someone who is 60 years or older. They are people who have several years on them and lots of life experience. They're most likely retired or semi-retired or volunteering their time. They're probably still active and having fun with friends and family. They do a lot of traveling. These are mature adults. They are NOT geriatric!

While you can have a mature adult who is in a geriatric condition, it's not true that all mature adults are geriatric. Most people who could be considered geriatric are in the later stages of life. As people get older, the chances of them having more health and physical problems increases. So, you may do some geriatric massage with mature adults, but most mature adults will not be looking for a true geriatric massage.

The following sections will help you understand the differences between a geriatric massage and a massage for a mature adult.

Geriatric Massage

Geriatric massage is a very specialized type of massage which was designed for people who are of advanced age and physically frail. Developed by Deitrich Miesler in 1982, this type of massage has techniques designed specifically for older, more frail, and more infirm clients. This type of massage is excellent for clients who have had a stroke, have Alzheimer's or severe Parkinson's, can't tolerate long times on a massage table (or can't even get on a massage table), or need very light pressure.

Geriatric clients will take more time and patience to get a session started and finished. These clients may not move quickly or easily. You may have a caregiver who will help the client prepare for the massage. Many times, when working with truly geriatric clients, you will have a shortened session of only 15 to 30 minutes. You may only have your client prone or supine, but not turn them over during the massage. Some clients may stay in a wheel chair or you may work work with them in their bed.

This type of massage is extremely beneficial to the truly geriatric client, but it will not do well for healthy and active mature adults.

As your mature adult clients age, you may end up doing more geriatric sessions, even if it's just a temporary situation due to an injury. Also, because you are working with mature adults, you will get calls from more people who might need a true geriatric session. If you plan to specialize in working with mature adults, it would be good to also get at least some training in geriatric massage so you will be ready for any situation that arises.

Massage for Mature Adults

Many times, a massage for a mature adult isn't much different from a massage you would give to someone who is 30, 40, or 50 year old. When you have a healthy mature adult, you won't have to adjust your massage at all. But, if you have a mature adult who is physically slowing down due to the aging process, you may need to start adjusting his or her massage a little bit. Eventually, you may even end up doing geriatric massage for that client when or if he or she reaches that stage. The main issue is that you have to be able to evaluate the client in front of you (see Chapter 5 for details).

I cannot judge the condition of my clients just by checking their date of birth. I have a 75-year-old client who looks for, and can handle, a 90-minute deep massage with firm pressure, but then I have another 75-year-old client who needs a 60-minutc light touch and enjoys a Swedish circulatory massage. It is my evaluation and communication with my client that helps me get a much better picture of what type of massage will most benefit my client. And that is the key to succeeding when working with mature adults.

For many mature adult clients your biggest adjustment will be pressure and comfort on the table. However, other clients will need more attention and adjustments to their session like a shorter session, a massage that takes place somewhere other than on a massage table, or avoiding certain areas. Chapter 6 provides information on common conditions you may run into when working with some mature adults.

As massage therapists working with mature adults, we need to remember that a person's age, gray hair, or wrinkles do not tell us what kind of health that person is in. Each client is an individual and we must adjust our techniques and session to what is best for the client on our table. For some mature adults, this can be a firm, deep massage, for others it will be a light circulatory massage.

I have heard stories from mature adults about a massage they had received in the past did not meet their needs. Either the therapist they saw used too much pressure, causing pain during the massage and bruises after the massage, or the therapist used very little pressure even though the client wanted it and could accept a firmer massage! Both were inappropriate for the respective clients. If these therapists had properly evaluated their clients before the massage, those clients would have been much happier! In the end, treating each person as the individual they are will help you work well with this growing population.

So, when you have a mature adult walk into your massage practice, keep in mind that you have to evaluate each client based on their body condition, not what you think based only on their age or appearance. Mature adults will appreciate your work a lot more when they know you are treating them as an individual with individual needs and not just assuming they are an "old" person who needs a light, shorter, geriatric massage.

Chapter 3 – Benefits of Massage

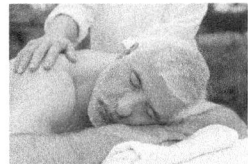 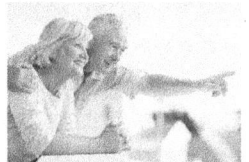 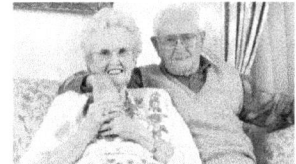

Massage has become a more accepted and available health option for everyone and mature adults are no different. While everyone can enjoy and benefit from massage, mature adults will benefit even more.

Today's mature adults are healthier and more active than their predecessors. When they retire they don't just settle into a comfy chair and wile away the day watching TV. They are out working part time, volunteering, playing sports, working out, getting together with friends, and traveling. While being active helps to keep people young at heart and helps them to stay active longer, they still must deal with the effects of getting older.

This chapter provides information on how massage can help with some specific effects of aging.

Benefits of Massage

As we get older, we lose muscle mass and flexibility, circulation to our hands and feet decreases, and our joints can become stiff either from over or under use. Remaining active helps reduce some of the effects of these aging problems. Massage can further reduce the effects of aging and will also help with any negative effects of being active, such as overworking muscles.

For older people who are not as active as their on-the-go counterparts, whether from choice, injury, or illness, massage can be just as important, if not more so. When muscles are not used regularly, they atrophy or become tense and sore because they are stuck in the same position for a long time. Massage will help these muscles get movement and blood flow, which will help them move and feel better.

Regardless of the activity level of a mature adult, massage can offer the following benefits:
- improved circulation
- improved range of motion, mobility, and flexibility
- relief from muscle tension, soreness, and fatigue

- reduced stress, anxiety, and pain
- improved concentration, balance, and posture
- movement of muscles and joints that may not get moved otherwise

Improved Circulation

The cardiovascular system includes the heart, circulatory, and lymphatic systems. The system circulates blood, allowing oxygen and nutrients to be delivered throughout the body.

As we age, blood flow can be hampered due to things such as:
- a buildup of plaque
- a reduction of elasticity in the vascular tissue
- unresolved stress

The lymphatic system is an important tool for waste removal and helps with the immune response. Wastes that are removed through the lymphatic system include:
- excess fluid
- pathogens
- dead blood cells
- toxins
- cells affected with cancer

Massage improves circulation by doing the following:
- helping blood to flow better
- bringing fresh oxygen and nutrients to the tissues
- getting rid of metabolic waste that builds up in muscles after activity by moving it into lymphatic circulation

- reducing arterial blood pressure through lymphatic circulation

Improved Range of Motion, Mobility, and Flexibility

As people age, their joints can become stiff. Overuse or injuries to joints when someone is younger can cause joints to become stiff as they age or allow arthritis to develop. Because of this, they may not move as much as they get older and this in turn, can cause even more joint stiffness!

Massage, with its warming effects can soothe under- and over-used joints, allowing people to move more freely.

Relief from Muscle Tension, Soreness, and Fatigue

Just like everyone else, mature adults can get muscle tension, soreness, and fatigue. This can result from either an active or sedentary lifestyle. Many mature adults still participate in sports, do work in and around the house, move furniture, or just about anything else younger folks do! For mature adults who are more sedentary, this lack of movement can cause tension and soreness due to consistent pressure being applied to the same area for an extended period of time.

Muscular issues can also stem from medicines your client is taking. If your client is only on a medication that causes muscular soreness for a short time, you can help them through the tough spell, but if they are on the medication for an extended period of time, you will be a much-needed part of their overall health plan. People in chronic pain face not only the physical, but emotional toll of constant pain.

Massage warms up connective tissue, relaxes muscles, and helps to work out knots and tension areas. Specific massage techniques can also help to reduce or even eliminate adhesions in muscle tissue, which can also cause tension and soreness.

Whatever the cause of muscle problems, massage can help relieve muscle tension, soreness, and fatigue for your mature adult clients.

Reduced Stress, Anxiety, and Pain

Getting older can be rough. A person may not be sure if their money will last for the rest of their life. They may be dealing with health issues or the death of a spouse. Sometimes dealing with difficult family relations can cause stress or anxiety. They may feel out of touch or that today's world moves too fast and they are being left behind.

The above issues do not affect all mature adults, but for those who face these issues, even if for a short time, massage can be a comfort in their life. Massage provides healing touch and lets clients know that they are not alone in the world.

Improved Concentration, Balance, and Posture

Poor concentration can be caused by anxiety, depression, insomnia, and fatigue. Massage can help with these issues and, therefore, may help with poor concentration.

Balance

Balance issues can be a big problem for older adults. When a person is dizzy or unsteady on their feet, they have an increased chance of falling, which can cause injury. Balance issues can be caused by:

- medications
- ear infections
- head injuries
- low blood pressure
- problems that affect skeletal or visual systems

A 2012 study (Sefton, Yarar, and Berry) showed that a single 60-minute full-body massage had a stabilizing effect on static and dynamic balance and physiological factors related to stability in older adults.

Posture

Over time, bad posture can take its toll. For mature adults, a lifetime of poor posture can cause serious problems in terms of pain and mobility. While it can be difficult to totally reverse 30, 40, or 50 years of bad posture effects, massage can help relieve some postural problems in older adults. Also, depending on the age of the client and how long a problem has existed, you may even be able to correct some postural problems, but it will take time.

If it is too late to correct a postural problem, you can still provide relief to your mature adult clients by relaxing muscles that are under stress due to such problems. This muscle relaxation can help to open up your client's chest (possibly helping them to breathe better) and may help them to stand up straighter.

Movement of Muscles and Joints that May Not Get Moved Otherwise

For mature adult clients who are more sedentary due to injury or physical condition, massage can be a great way to activate and move underused muscles and stiff joints that may not otherwise get moved.

Passive stretches and range of motion techniques will engage underused muscles and enable joint activity. This movement will help to increase circulation to these areas, increasing blood flow and nourishing the muscles. Joints will have freer movement. Massage strokes will also provide stimulation for underused muscles.

Chapter 4 – Getting Started

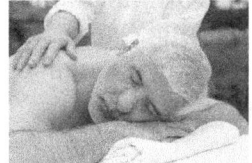 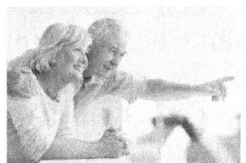 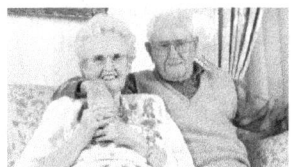

Massage is an excellent way for mature adult clients to stay active and healthy as they age and get relief from the effects of aging. The massage therapist who works with this population has the opportunity to make great improvements in their clients' lives, maybe even more so than when working with many younger clients.

However, as we discussed earlier, a mature adult can be anywhere from 60 to 100 plus years old and there is a LOT of room for different health conditions in that age range. So, while many mature adult clients won't need any special treatment when compared to someone who is 30, 40, or 50 years old, there are many for whom you will have to make adjustments.

Some of these adjustments will be minor, others will be much bigger and will be more in the area of a geriatric massage. It is important for you to know and be aware of possible issues you may face when working with mature adults. This chapter discusses the issues and considerations you MAY face when working with mature adults.

Cautions

Although massage is very beneficial for mature adults, some precautions must be taken when working with this group. In my experience, age is not necessarily the indicator of what precautions I must take when giving a massage to a mature adult. I have several clients in their 70s who benefit from a firm, deep massage and other clients in their 70s with whom I have to use a much lighter touch. As with any massage, the therapist must make a determination of what type of massage techniques should be used and how much pressure to use with any given client, keeping in mind that firm pressure to one client is medium or light to others. Some things to keep in mind when working with mature adult clients include:
- their skin may be thinner
- they may have less muscle mass
- their bones may be more fragile

- they may have less flexibility
- they may have pacemakers
- they may have had hip or knee replacements
- they may be taking medications that can be affected by massage
- they may have major health problems

It is important that you learn to evaluate your mature adult client (see Chapter 5 for details). You may need to take a little extra time during your intake interview to fully understand what's going on with your client. Although many mature adult clients will not require major scrutiny, you will need to be prepared for those clients who do.

One of the main reasons you apply caution is so that you give the appropriate massage to your client. For an older, more frail person, firm pressure may hurt or bruise them. But, many mature adults can take that pressure and WANT it. They don't want to get a "light" massage.

It can be tough to remember to adjust your pressure if you're going from heavier work to lighter work in the same day (or if you've done a lot of heavier work several days in a row). Always make sure you keep in mind the needs and wants of the body you are working on and stay present in your work.

One other consideration to keep in mind when working with mature adults is to stay away when you are sick. As people get older, it is harder to fight off illness and usually takes longer to recover. If you even think you might be coming down with something, you are probably better off to reschedule an appointment than take that sickness to your client. He or she will appreciate it!

The 4 Cs

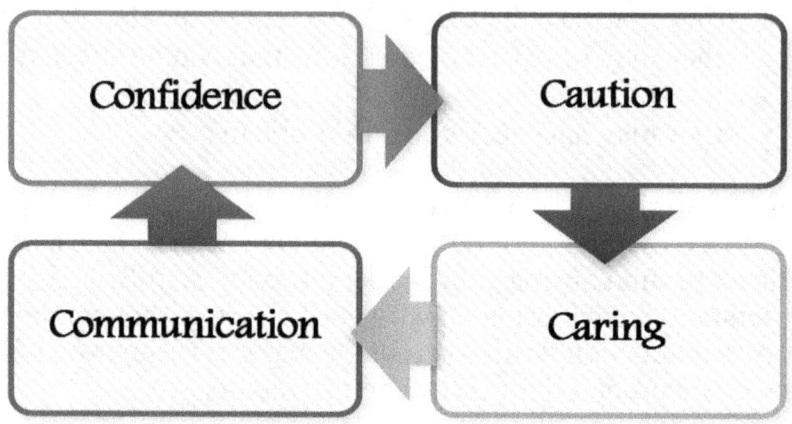

The 4 Cs

When I designed my original Massage for Seniors CE course (now Massage for the Mature Adult), I came up with the 3 Cs of working with seniors. I felt that these three things were the guidelines to working with seniors. The three Cs were confidence, caution, and communication. It recently occurred to me, though, that I had left a C out! That fourth C was caring. If you keep the 4 Cs in mind while you are working with mature adults, you will do very well. The following sections will discuss these guidelines in detail.

Confidence

You always want to show confidence when you are doing an intake interview and working with your mature adult client. This is not arrogance or a feeling that you know better than your client. It is a belief that you understand how to do massage and what you can and can't do. If you don't have an outward appearance of confidence, your client will not trust you and with mature adults, trust is paramount (we will discuss trust more later on in this chapter).

Even when you run into a situation that is new or different for you (and you will), you can't get flustered or let the situation overwhelm you. Even if inside your head you're thinking "Oh no! What do I do now?????" you need to have an outward appearance of calm and show confidence that you can handle the situation.

I once showed up at a client's home assuming that we would do a normal table massage. However, he informed me when I arrived that he could not do a table massage due to incontinence issues. This was the first time I had run into this situation! So, we went to his bedroom and I found a bench at the end of his bed. He was able to sit on the end of the bench and I could work on his back and neck while straddling and sitting on the bench behind him. Then I moved around him to do his arms, legs, and feet. This allowed me to give him his massage while giving him the ability to get up quickly if necessary.

I had another client who had a respiratory disease that required her to be constantly on oxygen. Again, this was a totally new experience for me. Although my client could get on a massage table, she could not lie prone and had some trouble lying supine. So, I did some side-lying work and when she was supine I propped her up with a couple of pillows. I also had to make sure I didn't step on her oxygen line during the massage. Each new session required an evaluation of how my client was doing that day, so each session was handled a little differently, but I always kept my head and figured out what was needed that day.

The two examples above were surprises for me when I walked into the clients' homes. But I didn't panic, and I found ways to work with my clients so they could get the massages they needed.

Especially if you haven't worked with older folks a lot, you will also run into medical and physical conditions that you haven't dealt with before. Chapter 6 gives you a brief overview of common conditions you may encounter, but you should also do your own research.

Most of the time you will learn about your client's issues when they first contact you. If you are not familiar with a condition, research it before you even go to the client's home so you will have an idea of what to expect and some initial ideas on how to proceed with your massage session.

Do your research before hand, but even if you get surprised by something, know that you can work out almost any situation. Just be ready to go with the flow!

Caution

Although you want to be confident, you also need to exercise caution with your mature adult client. Listen to what your client tells you. If you hear anything that raises a red flag, take some more time to get more information. Sometimes a client will be able to give you enough information about their condition that you will feel comfortable proceeding with the massage. However, there will be times when you will need to do more research.

If you are talking to a potential client on the phone, get as much information as possible during that first call. Then you can do some research on what the client told you to be prepared for your appointment. If you have a smart phone and you are already with your client, you can also look up information right there. A client will appreciate you taking the time to research their condition to make sure you won't harm him or her.

If the client can't give you the information you need and your research doesn't give you enough information for you to feel comfortable giving your client a massage, you may need to postpone the massage until your client has checked with their health care provider. You may also want clearance from a doctor if your research turns up potential contraindications (See Doctor's Approval below for more details).

The last thing you want to do is harm your client because you didn't ask questions or because you rushed ahead without enough information. Most clients will understand that it is their best interest you have in mind.

Communication

Communication is your number one tool when working with any client, but especially a mature adult client. If you don't know how your client is feeling or what's going on with them you could end up hurting them.

Check in with your client to make sure he or she is comfortable on the table and that the pressure is good for them. Although many mature adults reach a point where they have no trouble telling you if they don't like what you are doing, some may be more reticent. Remember, they may see you as the expert and not want to question you or they may think that a massage is supposed to hurt to do good.

Make sure you know that your client is happy with what you are doing. Especially with new clients, I like to check in about three times in a session. You don't want to over do it, but you should make sure all is good often enough that your client has a chance to speak up if necessary.

I had a client I had been massaging for a couple years and I had thought that I was giving her as much pressure as she wanted. She always complimented me on my massage. During a conversation one day, however, I found out that she could take and WANTED more pressure! So I communicated with her during our next appointment to make sure I gave her the pressure she wanted and she was much happier with the results!

Also check on temperature. If you're like me, you become hot while doing massages because of the physical labor involved. You may be sweating, but your client is chilly. I always carry a blanket with me, even in the heat of the Texas summers. I had one client who used to keep her house around 80 degrees and she still wanted a blanket!

You may also have to explain how the session will proceed each time you see a client. For clients who are getting older and whose mental faculties are slowing down, you may always need to remind them if you want to start them face down or face up and to get under the top sheet. Just be patient and give them the information again!

Of course, the most important part of getting feedback from your client is to address it. If it is a change that can be made without any problems, then do it! Don't ignore what the client tells you (I shouldn't have to say that, should I?). There may be times, however, when you will have to tell your client that you can't do what they want. In those instances, you need to tell them WHY you can't do it. For example, if your client has osteoporosis in her spine and she asks you to give her more pressure on her back, you are going to have to tell her you can't do it because you could cause a fracture. Most people will understand and be glad you knew enough to avoid doing them harm.

Always make sure you are communicating with your clients and giving them the massage that they want and need. The more your communicate, the more you will know and the happier your client will be!

Caring

Caring is one of the most important things you need when working with mature adults. If you don't care for your client, if you don't have empathy for your client, if you don't have patience, please don't work with mature adults. It frustrates me to no end when I hear how some mature adults are treated by other health care professionals or even some massage therapists. Remember, these are human beings and they deserve your caring, understanding, and patience.

You may run into clients who have a lot of health issues that they will tell you about. Many of those issues you will not be able to help with massage. I find it frustrating at times because I really wish I had a magic wand and could make all their aches and pains go away. I wish I could give them the body of a 20-year-old again. Unfortunately, I can't do that and I've come to accept it. But I still listen and try to help them in any way I can. I don't dismiss their complaints by saying things like "Well, that's just because you're old!"

It's hard to believe that someone would make such a blatant statement as the one above, and usually people don't. But, they will, however, say it in other ways that may not be as obvious, but are still dismissive. We need to remember that just because someone is older it doesn't mean that we can't help them feel better or even fix a problem. We may not be able to fix everything, but hopefully we can at least give our mature adult clients some relief.

Caring for your client also means being more attentive. Make sure your client can get on and off the table without any problems and if they do need help, offer it. If they require more than a steadying hand, get help from a spouse or caregiver unless you feel confident you can properly assist them (make it clear with family and caregivers of clients who need more help than you can provide in a session, that it is not your job to move the client, dress them, etc.). Be aware of any working signs that might indicate your client is uncomfortable and check in with them to see if you need to make any adjustments.

Also understand that unexpected health issues with your client or their spouse may cause your client to cancel an appointment at the last minute. Be understanding when this happens. Most mature adults are excellent at keeping appointments, but sometimes things happen. Care enough for your clients to be understanding when unfortunate incidents happen.

Doctor's Approval

For most of your mature adult clients, you will not need a doctor's approval to do your massage. This may be more of an issue when working with geriatric clients, but for the majority of mature adults this is not an issue.

However, there may be times when your mature adult client is having a procedure performed or is having a problem that has not yet been diagnosed, and that may give you pause. In such circumstances you will want to get a doctor's approval before doing the massage. Most clients will understand that this is for their own good and will appreciate that you do not want to do them harm.

Often, your client will have already talked to their doctor or physical therapist about massages and they may be able to tell you that the doctor or physical therapist thinks it is a good idea to continue the massage. You will have to decide if you want a specific note from the health care provider to put in your files. Especially if you're working with a new client, you may want to get one, just to protect yourself.

Once your mature adult client has spoken to their doctor, follow any guidelines given. Most times it might just be a need to wait a few weeks before getting a massage, or they may not be able to lay in a certain position for a specific period of time. Once you know your boundaries, you will be able to give your client the massage they need.

Where to Perform the Massage

Where you perform the massage for a mature adult client is not terribly important. Most active and healthy mature adults can come to your studio without much problem. If your mature adult clients have mobility issues or other problems that limit them getting out of the house, in-home (outcall) massage may be the best option.

I've have actually found that in-home massage is a great option for my mature adult clients. Some of my clients absolutely need me to come to them. Others just love the convenience and the fact they don't have to deal with traffic before and after a massage.

Truly geriatric clients will probably need you to come to them more often than not and that may mean working in their homes, in an assisted living facility, a nursing home, or even in a hospital.

If you are doing work somewhere other than your studio or your client's home, you may need to check in with the facility staff when you come and go or sign a log book. For nursing homes or hospitals, you may want to check with the facility to see if there are any specific requirements or procedures you need to follow when visiting your client.

Working with the Family/Caregiver

If you are working with a mature adult who is more in a geriatric condition, it will probably be necessary for you to interact more with family members and caregivers. These people will be great sources of information for you, especially if your client is having trouble communicating.

The important thing to remember when dealing with these types of situations is that you still must address your client. When you are establishing how the client is that day and how the session should proceed, a family member or caregiver may be the one doing most of the talking. Although you need to address and acknowledge this person, you MUST also include your client in the conversation. Do NOT talk only to the caregiver and ignore your client. As much as possible, bring your client into the conversation.

You will also experience the family dynamic and how caregivers work with your client. For the most part, it is best to stay out of any conflicts and keep your opinions to yourself. I've seen wonderful caregivers and spouses who really care for my clients. I've also seen situations that are less than ideal, but not elder abuse. Fortunately, I've never encountered a case of elder abuse. If you ever run into a situation that looks like it could be elder abuse, you should report it immediately. Hopefully, you will never encounter such a situation.

Medications

You do need to have some awareness of what medications your client is taking. Many medications will not affect how you do your massage, but some may affect when you do your massage so you may have to schedule the massage before or after the client takes the medication.

Topical medications are now used quite often. It is very important that we use caution if our clients have a topical medication patch. While you can massage around the patch, do not massage over it (it will come loose). You also don't want to touch the patch, especially on the side that contacts your client's skin. If you touch the side with the medication, you can get a dose of medication that was not meant for you!

If you use caution when working in and around a topical medication path, you should be fine.

Trust

Mature adults are an interesting group of people. On one hand, they have a lot of life experience and many have lead extremely interesting lives. Many were confident and big decision makers in their families and careers. Some mature adults still have that confidence that comes from a lifetime of living. However, as people get older, especially if they feel their mental faculties are slipping, they lose some of that confidence and they start to rely on others more and more.

It is important that you understand, appreciate, and honor the trust that some mature adult clients may place in you. They expect that what you are doing is appropirate for them. You are the expert when it comes to massage. But that expertise credit may also slip to other areas in their life as well.

I often get asked questions about health and medication issues or exercise or diets or various other tings a client may be considering or struggling with. It's important that we make sure we operate within our scope of practice and not lead our clients astray. I feel badly sometimes that I can't answer a client's question and I know they don't want to call the doctor's office to get the answer they need, but that is really the best way to handle their question. Many times, we will have a better relationship with our clients than they will have with their doctors or sometimes even their family. As a result, your clients may feel like they trust your opinion on an issue more than someone else.

Please don't abuse the trust a mature adult puts in you. Help them within the boundaries of your license and encourage them to check with others on things you are not qualified to answer.

Chapter 5 – Evaluating the Mature Adult Client

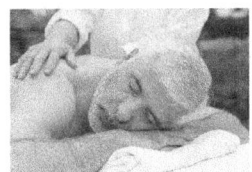 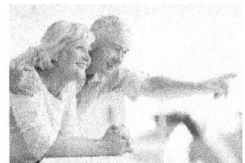 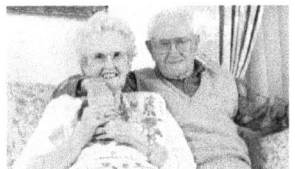

Many people, massage therapists included, see someone with wrinkles and white or gray hair and immediately think they need to treat that person with kid gloves. They assume the person may be frail and/or mentally slower due to old age. When it comes to massage, they may think that they can't do a full body massage, or they will have to use significantly less pressure, or only do a short session. However, this is often not the case.

Many mature adults have white or gray hair. But that doesn't mean that they're ready for the rocking chair at the old folks home! Today's mature adults are active and healthy. For many people, 60 is not old any more. They are still active in their community. They still play sports like tennis, pickle ball, and golf. They travel the world. If you suggested that they should only have a 20 or 30 minute massage session, they would laugh you out of the room!

Having said that, there are mature adults who do need more customized treatment. They lie somewhere between a hale and hearty mature adult and a geriatric client, but changes have begun to happen to their body as they have aged so some changes to the session may be needed. They may still be good with a full hour or hour and a half session, but you may need to adjust your pressure or use more lubricant. You may need to do a side-lying massage. Your client's flexibility may be impaired. They might have had hip or knee replacements. They may have a pacemaker. Their bones can be more brittle. None of these things absolutely prevents you from doing a full massage session.

So, how do you know how to treat and work with the mature adult who is in front of you? You have to evaluate that person as you would any other client, and understand what they have going on with their body. Once you have an idea of what is going on with the mature adult you are working with, the better you will be able to design a session that will be just what they wanted.

You will also want to look at how your client stands or sits. Are they steady on their feet? Is your client using a walker or is he or she still active and healthy? Do the client's limbs look strong and firm, or thin and frail?

Take the time to get to know your mature adult client and then you can create a session plan that will be beneficial as well as safe and comfortable. If you meet the needs of your mature adult clients, you will have the most dedicated clientele available!

The following sections discuss some key evaluation tools and considerations for mature adults.

Client Intake

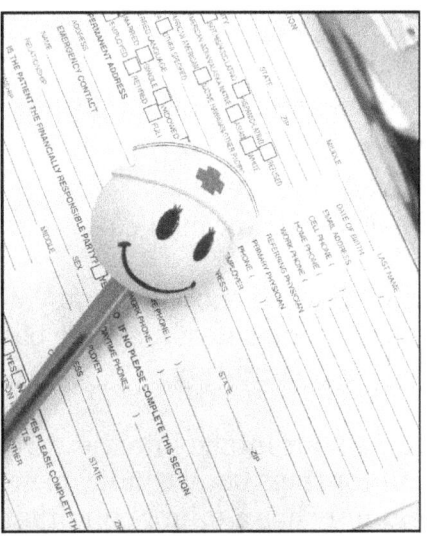

Intake Form

The first time you meet with your mature adult client, you will want to get a good understanding of what medical conditions (if any) they have and what they are looking to achieve in their sessions. For some of your clients, there might not be a lot to learn. For others, though, there may be a lot you need to learn before proceeding with the massage.

When you take a detailed client intake you will learn things like:
- whether your client has a pacemaker
- have they had any recent surgeries
- have they had any recent injuries
- do they have skin problems that would require you to use a different (or more) lubricant
- do they have any areas you need to avoid due to:
  - contraindications
  - injury
  - skin issues
- have they been having trouble sleeping
- do they have high blood pressure
- do they have heart problems
- do they have any major medical conditions

Basically, you want to learn enough about your client so you can give them the best and safest massage based on their needs, wants, and body condition.

While you are doing your intake interview, you also need to evaluate the client for their body condition and energy level. Even if your client only has a minor condition or issue that won't require you to make any major changes to how you do your massage, you want to know as much as possible before you start.

This is the time when you might learn something that may make you exercise some caution. Dig for more information if you are unfamiliar with a condition or you know that something a client has told you may cause a potential problem if you do the massage. The intake interview you do with your client will give you the information you need to do a safe and effective massage for your client.

Types of Massage

Properly evaluating your mature adult client during the client intake will help you make informed decisions about the type of massage you perform for your client. Some modalities (such as deep tissue) may not be suitable for a more frail client or a client with a specific condition, but for a strong, healthy mature adult client, almost anything is possible.

Depending on the comfort level of your client, if your client is on your massage table, you may only be able to do massage in the supine position, or the prone position. Or side-lying may be the best position for your client. If your client has a hyperkyphosis (Dowager's hump), you may need to put a pillow under your client's head when they are in the supine position. The important thing is to make sure your client is comfortable so they can relax and enjoy their massage, and you can do the work you need to do.

Working with mature adults requires you to adapt when necessary. You may walk into an appointment (with a new or existing client) thinking it's going to be a normal massage and find out you need to make a quick change such as doing a seated massage instead of a table massage.

If you are working with a more frail client, you may need to adjust your massage for a non-table setting. Perhaps you'll work with your client in a seated position. This can be in a wheelchair or scooter, or on a bench, or even in a regular chair.

Sometimes, you might even be able to use a massage chair to do your massage. Just make sure that your client can get in and out of the chair and that they are comfortable.

If you are using a massage chair, it may be hard for your client to move their legs into the correct position. Depending on your chair, you may be able to remove the knee pads to allow your client to keep their feet flat on the floor during the chair massage. If you can't remove the knee pads, your client may still be able to sit with their feet on the floor.

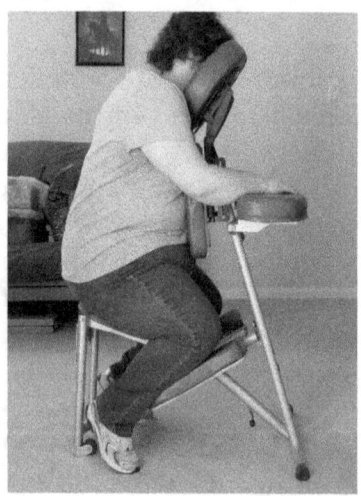

Client in Chair with Knee Pads

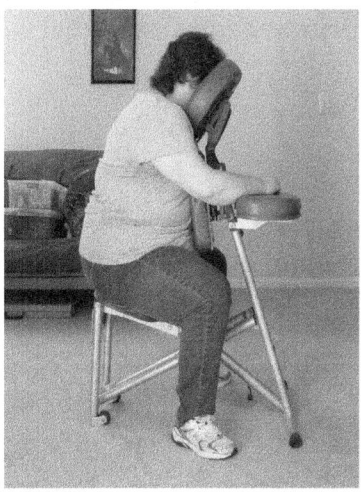

Client in Massage Chair without Knee Pads

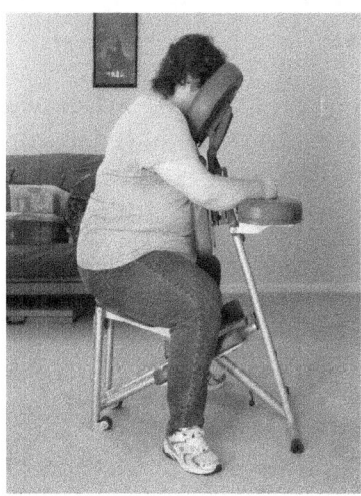

Client in Massage Chair Straddling Knee Pads

Whatever type of massage you decide is best for your mature adult client, your primary concern is that they are comfortable.

Skin Condition

As people age, their skin goes through physiological changes. It will lose water content and become dry and thin and can eventually take on a papery consistency. All of these conditions require the massage therapist to use a little caution when working with this type of skin.

When you have a client with thin or very dry sky, you will want to use more lubrication so that you have more glide. If you don't have enough lubrication, your strokes can hurt the client or even rip their skin, even if you're not using a lot of pressure. Also, the skin will soak up more of your lubrication, so you might have to apply it more often.

I recommend using a cream lubrication because it is easy to work with and soaks into the skin nicely, providing some hydration for your client's skin. Several of my clients have asked where they can get my cream because they like how it feels on their skin.

You may also have to be careful not to cause bruising when working with a client who has thinner skin. Remember that they won't have as much protection and a grip or touch that you think isn't too hard, may be too much for your client.

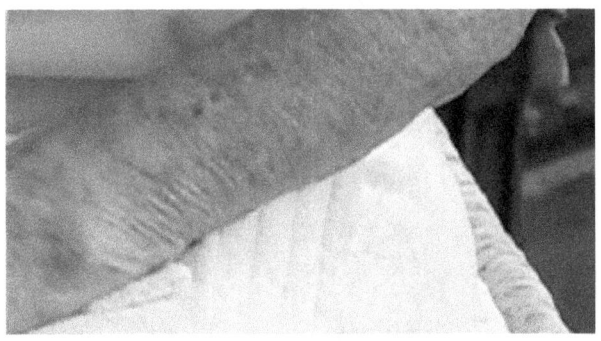

Dry/Thin Skin

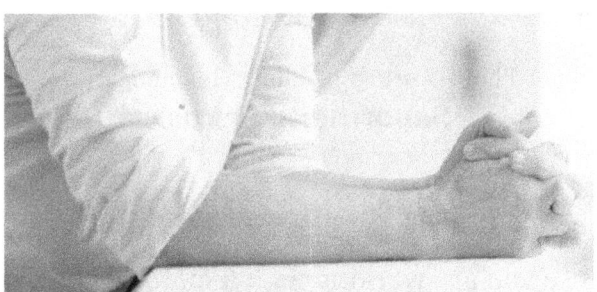

Well-Hydrated Skin

Of course, you may have mature adults who have very youthful and well-hydrated skin. In these cases, you won't have to make any adjustments at all.

A common skin condition you may run into is Seborrheic Kerstosis. Usually you will find these raised, brown spots on your client's back. Some clients only have a few of these, others can have a LOT! There are no contraindications for this condition so you can proceed with your massage as normal. Your client's back may be more "textured", but there will be no harm to you or your client if you massage over these spots.

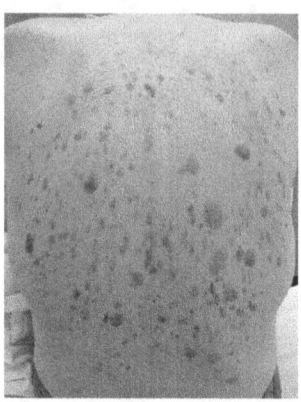

Photo courtesy of James Heilman, MD
Seborrheic Kerstosis

Pressure

Just because you are working with a mature adult, it does not mean that you should automatically lighten up your pressure. I have clients in their 70s and 80s who look for firmer pressure and enjoy a deep massage.

Of course, when you're talking about pressure, there are two things to consider. First, what does "firm" pressure mean to your client? Regardless of age, one person's firm is another person's light and vice verse. This is why this chapter is so important and why you need to understand how to evaluate the client before you. In a way, you have to interpret what your client is telling you so you understand what they need.

When a client says he or she wants a firm massage, it may be because they have a certain problem area they want worked out. Or, it could mean that they have gotten really light massages in the past and didn't feel satisfied with that. Or maybe a friend told them that a deep massage is the only type of "good" massage! Ask follow up questions to make sure you understand what it is your client is really looking for.

The second thing to consider is, can your clients handle the pressure they are asking for. Most mature adults, especially on the older, more frail side, have a good idea of what they can handle pressure-wise. They don't want to be hurt and so they will tell you they want lighter work. Sometimes, though, they will tell you that they want a deep tissue massage because someone they know told them that's what they needed. However, they have never had a deep tissue massage before and aren't prepared for what this type of massage is like. In these cases, it is up to you as the massage professional to explain what that type of work entails and that you think other techniques may be better for them.

It is also imperative to remember that even if your 75 year old client likes a firm, deep massage, it is still probably not the same firm, deep massage you would give to a 20 year old athlete! It's all relative. A good rule of thumb is to start out a little lighter than you think necessary and then work with your client, by asking them how the pressure is, to get to the correct pressure.

This is one of those times when communication between you and your client is imperative. Check in with your client to make sure the pressure is what they are looking for.

Posture

The posture of your client will tell you a lot about their physical condition. If you client has any postural deviations (see Chapter 8), more than likely they will have muscle tension and perhaps pain in the areas affected by the deviations. Because these deviations have probably been around for a long time, you may not be able to correct them, but you can help the client feel better for a period of time. However, if you have a mature adult who has a newer postural deviation, you may be able to work out those issues to correct the problem altogether.

I had a client who was in her mid-60s and her left hip was higher than her right hip. We spent several sessions with me massaging the entire body, but focusing on the hip area and trying to even out her hips. After ten sessions we were able to even out her hips and the changes have stayed in place since! If the client hadn't received the massage, her problem may have gotten worse, causing her more pain.

If your client has a postural deviation, you will also have to think about your client's comfort when on the table. For example, if your client has a hyperkyphosis, your client may not be comfortable laying in the supine position without a pillow under her head.

Depending on the specific problem, you may decide to do side-lying massage or even a seated massage, if lying on the table is not comfortable for your client. For most cases, client comfort on the table is your primary goal.

Range of Motion

When working with your mature adult clients, remember that their range of motion in their limbs may not be as full as a that of a younger person. Be careful and move slowly when moving legs and arms to make sure you don't push or pull a limb too far and cause the client pain.

Depending on how limited the client's range of motion is, you may not be able to move some limbs and you'll have to modify your massage strokes and techniques to address particular limbs differently.

Balance

As people get older, they can become unsteady on their feet. Sometimes this is a temporary condition caused by a medication or infection, or a longer term problem caused by issues such as peripheral neuropathy.

When a client is unsteady on their feet, you will have to use more caution with your client. You will want to make sure that they can get on and off the table without any problems. If they do not have a caregiver at hand, you may want to stay close until you know they have their feet under them and are steady before you leave the room.

Especially for a client who has balance issues, I would recommend that you end your session with the client in the supine position as opposed to the prone position. Being prone can cause disorientation when getting up, so it is better to end with your client face up.

You will also want to make sure to clean any lubrication from your client's feet before they get up, especially if they are going to be on a hard surface, to avoid the possibility of your client slipping and falling.

Energy Level

If your client's energy level is low, you may want to reduce the amount of time for your massage. This will be a decision you will make in conjunction with what else you know about your client. If your client is just a little tired that is one thing, but if your client's physical energy level is very reduced due to illness or recovery from surgery, a shorter session is a wise choice, especially if you are doing more gentle, relaxing work.

Wheelchair, Scooter, or Seated Massage

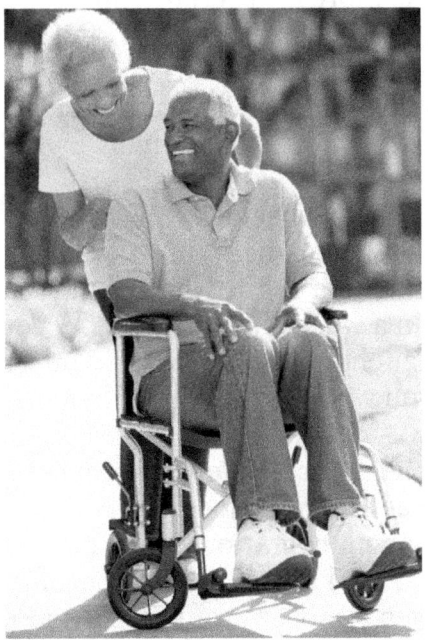

Mature Adult in Wheelchair

A client in a wheelchair or scooter can present some challenges. In this situation, you need to know if the client can get on and off a massage table without help. If they cannot and require a good deal of help, you should request that a loved one or caregiver be available to help. If the client just needs a hand to steady them or someone to move the chair or scooter out of the way, then you can handle that on your own.

If your client is wheelchair bound, either temporarily or permanently, you can still do some great work to help your client feel better. Obviously a full table massage is out. You will have to do your massage with your client in their chair or scooter. This gets more into geriatric massage, but you will focus on your client's neck, shoulders, and upper back. If the client is able to lean forward, you can do a little work on their lower back as well. Arms, lower legs, and feet can also be massaged with a client in a wheelchair.

If your client isn't in a wheelchair, but cannot do a full table massage, you can do massage with your client in a seated position. This is similar to the wheelchair scenario, but your client won't be in a wheelchair. Your client could sit on a stool, in a regular chair, or on a bench. You will focus on the same areas as you would with a client in a wheelchair.

Being in a wheelchair or scooter can be a temporary condition, such as after a major surgery or illness, or could be a more permanent condition due to mobility issues or a condition such as Parkinson's. It is important to be ready for this situation even if most of your mature adult clients are hale and hearty and are not in wheelchairs or scooters.

Chapter 6 – Specific Medical Conditions

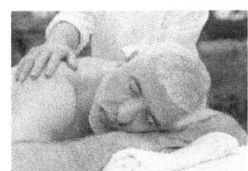 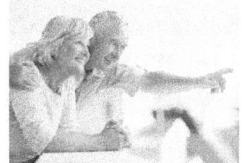 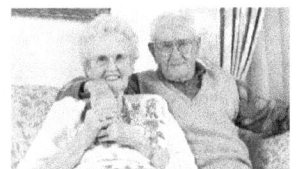

In this chapter I've provided an overview of some of the more common medical conditions you may encounter when working with mature adults. For more specific details on these conditions or ones not listed here, do your research. Check online sources, your pathology book, and, when necessary, discuss the client's medical condition with their health care team and/or doctor.

This chapter is not intended to be an exhaustive discussion of the medical conditions listed. It is meant to give you some basic information that will help guide you in determining if you need more information to proceed with a massage.

When you encounter a client with one of these conditions, or another condition not mentioned in this book, don't forget the 4 Cs discussed in Chapter 4. Always use caution, confidence, communication, and caring when working with your mature adult clients.

Some of the conditions listed in this chapter are more common in a geriatric massage setting, but you may run into clients with early stages of these conditions so I've included them. Also, if you decide to do geriatric massage as well, you will want to be knowledgeable about these conditions and this will give you a starting point.

This chapter mostly assumes Swedish and deep tissue modalities will be used. Practitioners of other modalities should do more research to see if their modality is supportive or contraindicated for that specific condition.

Specific Conditions

Alzheimer's Disease

NOTE: This condition is more commonly found when doing geriatric massage. However, you may run into mature adults who are in the early stages of this disorder. In the early stages, the type of massage you perform probably won't be much different from a regular massage. In the later stages, though, your massage can be vastly different.

Description

Alzheimer's disease (Alzheimer's) is the most common form of dementia. It is a progressive degenerative disorder of the brain causing memory loss, personality changes, and eventually, death. This disorder affects about five percent of the U.S. population and increases with age. Eleven percent of people over 65 have this condition and the prevalence doubles every five years after that. About one-third of those over 85 have Alzheimer's.

Massage Considerations

Massage does not slow or reverse the disease, but it can improve the quality of life of the client. An Alzheimer's client may become less disruptive, show better sense of orientation, and have more positive social interactions after a massage.

Keep in mind that the Alzheimer's client may have other conditions that may contraindicate massage, so check with the client's doctor before working with Alzheimer's clients. Also, the client may not be able to communicate clearly, so you will need to be able to interpret nonverbal signals. If the client feels agitated or unsafe at any time, you will need a caregiver nearby to address the issue. Having a caregiver nearby during the session is advisable.

Do not work from behind an Alzheimer's client. Always make sure your client can see you while you are working.

Amyotrophic Lateral Sclerosis (Lou Gehrig Disease)

NOTE: This condition is more commonly found when doing geriatric massage. However, you may run into mature adults who are in the early stages of this disorder. In the early stages, the type of massage you perform probably won't be much different from a regular massage. In the later stages, though, your massage can be vastly different.

Description

Amyotrophic Lateral Sclerosis (ALS) is a progressive neurodegenerative disease that destroys motor neurons in the central and peripheral nervous systems. This condition causes voluntary muscles to atrophy. In the final stages, the respiratory muscles that control breathing deteriorate to the point where the patient must be put on a respirator for the rest of their life.

There is no one specific cause of ALS. Only five to ten percent of cases in the U.S. are genetically linked. The average age of diagnosis is 55. Patients usually live two to ten years after diagnosis.

In the early stages of the disease, common symptoms include:
- minor leg or arm weakness
- trouble with speech or swallowing
- cramping and muscle pain

Massage Considerations

Massage can help ALS clients in the following ways:
- minimize pain and suffering
- prevent joints from becoming stiff through gentle massage and range of motion techniques

- increase circulation to help prevent the development of decubitus ulcers (bed sores) due to lack of activity
- overcome depression

Although massage can have benefits for ALS clients, you will need to make sure there are no other problems or conditions that would contraindicate massage. You should communicate with the client's health care team to make sure you are not causing harm.

Keep in mind that you will probably have to deal with muscle spasms and contractions during the massage. You may also not be able to easily communicate with the client during the massage.

Arthritis

There are two types of arthritis you will see, rheumatoid arthritis and osteoarthritis.

Rheumatoid Arthritis

Description

Rheumatoid arthritis (RA) is an autoimmune condition where the synovial membranes of joints are affected by immune system cells. It can also involve inflammation of tissues outside the musculoskeletal system. The disease often starts when a person is in middle age and more often in older adulthood, but younger people can also get it. It occurs more often in women than men.

Massage Considerations

With RA clients you should not work during an acute phase or flare up because it is an inflammatory condition. Circulatory massage would not be appropriate at this time. However, in the subacute phase, massage is helpful with relieving pain and improving mobility and the health of the tissue surrounding the joints. Work within the tolerance of your client. You goal in this type of massage is to relieve pain and inflammation and reduce stress.

Osteoarthritis

Description

Osteoarthritis (OA) is also known as degenerative joint disease (DJD) and is the most common form of joint disease. With this condition, the cartilage cushions between the joints break down. As we age, the water portion of the cartilage increases and the protein composition degenerates. This causes the cartilage to form tiny crevasses. The cartilage surfaces then fray, wear, ulcerate, and may wear away completely, which causes the joint to slide bone-on-bone, causing pain and limiting joint mobility. The main areas affected by OA include:
- knees
- hips
- spine
- hands

OA can occur in other joints, but the above four are the main ones affected.

Massage Considerations

Moderate to light pressure should be used during your sessions. Check in with your client to make sure the pressure is not too much. Most clients will find a gentle massage soothing to aching joints. Caution should be used if your client has any of the following:

- damaged or eroded joints
- flare up of inflammation, fever, or skin rash

According to the Arthritis Foundation, massage has the following benefits:

- improved function
- stress relief
- moderation of the immune system
- improved pain, stiffness, fatigue, anxiety, and depression

Balance Disorders

Description

Balance disorders are common in the older population. There can be many different reasons for balance issues including:

- medication effects
- peripheral neuropathy
- low blood pressure
- problems that affect skeletal or visual systems

Types of balance disorders include:

- labryinthitis – inflammation within the body or membranous labyrinth of the inner ear.

- acute vestibular neuropathy – damage to the vestibular portion of cranial nerve 8.
- Meniere's disease – episodes of vertigo along with tinnitus, hearing loss, and a feeling of fullness in the middle ear.
- head injury – blows to the head, violent sneezing, or whiplash-type accidents that cause inner ear fluid to break into the middle ear.
- benign paroxysmal positional vertigo (BPPV) – changes in position of the head (getting up, lying down, rolling over).

Massage Considerations

You will need to make sure clients can get on and off the table without injury and make sure your client has their balance once they get off the table and begins to walk. It is a good idea to end your massage with your client in the supine position because the prone position can add a sense of disorientation when getting up from a massage.

Bursitis

Description

Bursitis is an inflammation of the small sac (bursa) found inside joints. The bursae help ease the movement of tendons over bony angles and help cushion the bones where they would otherwise bang against each other. Bursitis usually occurs in larger joints such as the shoulder, hip, knee, or elbow and is usually caused by repetitive motions. This condition causes pain and limits mobility.

Symptoms include:
- aching and stiffness in joints
- limited range of motion
- swelling, redness, heat radiating from the joint (superficial only, not deep)
- pain with passive or active movement

A doctor's examination is usually needed to determine if the pain the client is feeling is from bursitis, a strain, or arthritis.

Note that bursitis can sometimes be caused by a bacterial infection, gout, or rheumatoid arthritis.

The condition comes in many varieties and locations. Some other names for bursitis include:
- housemaid's knee
- student's elbow
- weaver's bottom
- jack hammerer's shoulder

Massage Considerations

You should avoid massage in the acute phase of the condition. In the non-acute phase, you can work the area. Be careful not to irritate the bursae again by rubbing directly on the joint. You can sometimes address the muscles that cross over the affected joint, which may help decompress the bones that are irritating the bursae.

If the bursitis is caused by an infection, you should not do the massage.

Massage can help your client relax and reduce the amount of discomfort caused by the bursitis.

Cancer

There are many types of cancer. I've broken this section into two subsections, general and skin cancer. This book is not about oncology massage, but you will have mature adults with cancer issues so I wanted to include a brief description of the types of cancer that exist. Because we, as massage therapists, see a lot of our client's skin, I included a separate discussion of skin cancer.

If you want to work with clients with cancer on a more regular basis, you should get in-depth training in oncology massage so you can properly help your clients and understand the treatments they are receiving.

General

Description

Cancer is an uncontrolled replication of cells that turns into tumors. The tumors can then spread throughout the body through surrounding tissues.

There are many types of cancer. You should work with your client's health care team during your massage treatment of a client with cancer. Massage is not usually contraindicated just because a client has cancer, but you definitely want to know what you are doing!

Note that massage can NOT spread cancer. You should avoid massaging a solid tumor site, but the rest of the body can be massaged.

The following list gives you a brief description of several different types of cancer you might run into (either current treatment or post treatment) when working with mature adults.

- breast cancer – development of tumors in the epithelial or connective tissue of the breast. It is the second most frequently diagnosed cancer in women. Approximately 77% of patients are over 50 years old when diagnosed. You may have clients who have had breast reconstructive surgery or a single or double mastectomy. If your client has implants, make sure your client is comfortable when lying prone.
- lymphoma – cancer in the lymph nodes that involves a mutation of the DNA in specific white blood cells.
- liver cancer – hepatocellular carcinoma (primary liver cancer) is a cancer that originates in the liver. Secondary or metastatic liver disease results from cancer that originated in another part of the body and leads to tumors in the liver.
- lung cancer – growth of malignant cells in the lungs that can eventually form tumors. This type of cancer is very capable of spreading before tumors are detectable because there is easy access to the circulatory and lymph systems.
- myeloma – blood cancer that involves maturing B cells found in bone marrow.

- pancreatic cancer – begins as a mutation of certain genes that sponsor uncontrolled growth of cells in the pancreas. It usually grows in the exocrine ducts of the pancreas, but it can grow in endocrine-producing cells as well.
- prostate cancer – growth of malignant tumor cells in the prostate gland.
- stomach cancer – growth of malignant tumors in the stomach that can block the passage of food through the digestive system.
- skin cancer – see details in the Skin Cancer section below.

Massage Considerations

Massage helps to reduce stress and anxiety and can improve immune function. You need to have a clear understanding of what treatment your client is undergoing. Communication with your client's health care team is paramount.

If your client is undergoing chemotherapy and radiation, avoid deep massage and strong pressure. Also avoid touching any sensitive skin in the treatment area. If lymph nodes have been removed, only very light touch on the affected arm and around the underarm should be used. If your client has arm lymphedema, you should avoid the affected arm and underarm area completely unless you are trained in manual lymphatic drainage.

Skin Cancer

Description

Skin cancer is a common form of cancer and can be a minor or major issue depending on the type of cancer and when it is found.

Common forms of skin cancer include:
- actinic keratosis (precancerous lesions)
- basal cell carcinoma
- squamous cell carcinoma
- malignant melanoma

Actinic keratosis is precancerous lesions that can lead to squamous cell carcinoma. It can be identified as brown or red scaly lesions that usually appear on the forehead, tops of ears, hands, or other areas that get a lot of sun exposure.

Basal cell carcinoma is the most common type of skin cancer. It is slow-growing and is usually not dangerous as long as it is treated and not left to interfere with other tissues. Basal cell carcinoma can appear in several different ways. The most common versions include the following:
- nodular – small, hard lump with rounded edges and a soft, sunken middle.
- pigmented – looks like nodular, but the lesions are usually dark brown or black.
- superficial – can resemble eczema or psoriasis and appears in pink or reddish-brown patches.
- micronodular – multiple small, well-defined, yellowish white lesions.

- morpheaform (infiltrating) – looks like scar tissue on the surface of the skin.

Squamous cell carcinoma occurs in the middle layers of the epidermis due to a malignancy of keratinocytes. Because it can metastasize through the lymph system, it can be more dangerous than basal cell carcinoma. The squamous cell carcinoma tumors appear on preexisting lesions and areas where the skin has a long history of damage and repair. The sores appear and do not heal.

Malignant melanoma can start from a preexisting mole or in areas that have been exposed to the sun, but this is not always the case. Key features of melanoma include:
- asymmetrical – benign moles are usually circular or oval, but melanoma has an uneven shape.
- border – borders are irregular and may blend into the skin.
- color – multicolored with brown, black, and sometimes purple mixed together.
- diameter – large. More than 6 mm across should be referred to a doctor.
- elevated – can be elevated partly from the skin, but this is not always the case.

Massage Considerations

In general, most clients with skin cancer can be massaged. If there are any undiagnosed skin lesions, the client's doctor should be consulted. Any tumors should be avoided. If the client is undergoing any treatments such as surgery, skin grafts, irradiation, or chemotherapy, you should work with the client and their health care team to make sure any massage sessions will be beneficial and not harmful to the client.

Although it is out of the scope of practice for a massage therapist to diagnose a condition, if you see something suspicious on your client's skin, do mention it and suggest they see a doctor. You don't want to alarm your client, just make it clear you're not sure, but it would be better for them to have it checked. Most of your mature adults clients will appreciate your heads up.

Crohn's Disease

Description

Crohn's Disease is a progressive inflammatory disorder that can affect any part of the gastro-intestinal (GI) tract and disrupts normal digestion. It is not the same thing as ulcerative colitis, but both conditions are discussed under the umbrella term, inflammatory bowel disease. Diagnosis of this condition usually occurs in people aged 15 to 30 and then again when someone is over 55. Because it has periods of flare ups and remission, an autoimmune component is suspected.

Massage Considerations

Massage can be helpful during remission. During flare ups, your client may not be comfortable on the table. It is probably best to avoid deep abdominal work, but creating a parasympathetic response for increased efficiency of digestion and nutrient absorption can be helpful.

You will want to work with your client's doctor to get input on how best massage can help with this particular client's specific health issues and whether to avoid the abdomen or work lighter.

Decubitus Ulcers (Bed Sores)

NOTE: This condition is something you would find more when doing geriatric massage. When you are working with truly geriatric clients or clients who have been confined to a wheel chair or bed for a long period of time due to recovery from an illness, you may see this more often.

Description

Decubitus ulcers are open wounds on the skin and subcutaneous tissue caused by poor circulation due to prolonged pressure on body parts, especially bony protuberances. This condition is also known as bedsores, pressure sores, and trophic ulcers. It happens to bedridden patients, often in a hospital or nursing home setting. Most clients who get bedsores are 70 years or older. It is more common in those with fragile skin.

The most common places where bed sores appear are on the hips, back, ankles, and buttocks.

Massage Considerations

Locally contraindicated. Because the condition is caused by a lack of circulation, some circulatory work can be beneficial, but it should be done around the area with the sore, but not directly on the sore. Massage can better be used as a preventive measure.

Depression

Description

Depression is a central nervous system (CNS) disorder involving a genetic predisposition, chemical changes, and often a triggering event that results in a person losing the ability to enjoy life. It can be long-lasting, self-propagating, and debilitating and can affect almost any age. In mature adults, the symptoms can mimic or coexist with other specifically geriatric diseases. If depression occurs in a mature adult, presenting symptoms are likely to be physical rather than emotional and include headaches, back pain, and digestive comfort and they are unlikely to be recognized as signals for a major depressive disorder.

Massage Considerations

Massage can be very beneficial to a depressive person. It improves the hypothalamic-pituitary-adrenal (HPA) axis. It moves people from a sympathetic to a parasympathetic state, increasing serotonin secretion and decreasing cortisol, which creates a pleasurable experience that is good for your client.

Some cautions – if your client starts feeling better, he or she may want to stop taking their medication. You should not recommend this. The client should discuss any medication changes their doctor. If depression is caused by a traumatic event, you should not try to counsel your client. Refer them to a qualified therapist.

Diabetes Mellitus

Description

Diabetes Mellitus is a group of related disorders that result in hyperglycemia (elevated levels of sugar in the bloodstream). Type 1 and type 2 diabetes account for 98% of all diabetes diagnoses. A description of each type follows:

- Type 1 – insulin-dependent diabetes mellitus (IDDM). It is the less common type of diabetes and can be brought on by:
  - exposure to certain drugs and chemicals
  - a complication of another condition
  - some kinds of infections
- Type 2 – used to be called non-insulin-dependent (NDDM), but that is no longer accurate. It is the most common type of diabetes. 90% of people are obese when diagnosed. It can be controlled with diet, exercise, and sometimes anti-diabetes drugs. Eventually, most patients benefit from supplementing insulin.

Types of diabetic emergencies include:

- ketoacidosis – a critical shortage of insulin and lack of glucose in the cells of type 1 diabetics. Can be brought on by stress, infection, or trauma and can lead to shock, coma, and death. Only occurs in people with type 1 diabetes.
- hyperosmolar syndrome – causes a change in the pH of the blood. Related to high blood sugar in type 2 diabetics. Can lead to shock, coma, and death.
- insulin shock – too much insulin is circulating in the blood. It can be due to either too much insulin being

administered or an event such as a skipped meal, sudden exertion, stress, infection, or trauma which has resulted in the consumption of all available blood sugar (hypoglycemia). Symptoms include dizziness, confusion, weakness, and tremors. Can lead to coma and death if not treated quickly by ingesting juice, milk, candy, or sugared soda to replace blood sugar.

Complications of diabetes include:
- cardiovascular disease
- edema
- ulcers, gangrene, and amputations
- kidney disease
- impaired vision
- neuropathy

Massage Considerations

Massage can be helpful to many people with diabetes. Improved circulation can improve cell insulin uptake. Massage can help increase mobility and tissue elasticity that has been diminished due to a thickening of the connective tissue due to increased blood sugars.

Some people believe it is best to schedule massages when the client's insulin is not at its activity peak. The client may want to eat a small meal before getting a massage.

Blood glucose levels can change when receiving massage, so it is a good idea to have a source of sugar (juice, milk, candy, sugared sodas) close by in case the client's blood sugar drops (hypoglycemia) during the massage. Your client may carry

their own glucose tablets with them. Symptoms of hypoglycemia include:
- excessive sweating
- faintness or headache
- inability to wake up
- spaciness
- irritability
- change in personality
- rapid heartbeat

Be careful of clients with neuropathy caused by diabetes (see section Peripheral Neuropathy).

Disc Disease

Description

Disc disease is an umbrella term for a condition in which the nucleus pulposus and/or the annulus fibrosis extends beyond its normal borders. There may be pain if someone presses on the spinal cord or spinal nerve roots, but the client may have no symptoms.

Muscle tension can lead to injury and strain the spinal column, which can accelerate the onset of degenerative spine conditions.

A clear diagnosis from a medical professional is important because there are other conditions that can have similar symptoms to disc disease. Other conditions include spondylosis, irritated spinal ligaments (ligament sprains), and (rarely) bone tumors.

Disc problems can be discussed/described in the following terms:

- herniated nucleus pulposus – the nucleus pulposus extends beyond the posterior margin of the vertebral body. Damage can be of the following types:
  - bulge – the entire disc protrudes symmetrically beyond the normal boundaries of the vertebral body.
  - protrusion – the nucleus pulposus extends out of the annulus at a specific location.
  - extrusion – a small piece of the nucleus protrudes with a narrow connection back to the body of the nucleus.
  - rupture – the nucleus pulposus has burst and leaked its entire contents into the surrounding area.
- degenerative disc disease – small, cumulative tears of the annulus, along with decreased disc height and dehydration of the nucleus. Often considered a normal part of the aging process, but smoking, obesity, and a sedentary lifestyle can accelerate it. It is a degeneration of the annular fibers of the intervertebral disc.
- internal disc disruption – the nucleus protrudes through the annulus but stays within the boundaries of the whole disc. Often related to trauma in addition to cumulative degenerative disc disease.
- spondylosis – degenerative changes in the facet joints and eventual fusing of the joint capsules.
- lumbago – low back pain.
- sciatica – compression or inflammation of the sciatic nerve. Can be caused by disc herniation, vertebral osteophytes, or piriformis syndrome.

Massage Considerations

Massage can help relieve muscle tension that is contributing to your client's pain and discomfort. Check in with your client for level of pain or discomfort they have that day as well as when you are massaging them. Work to create space for the retreat of the bulging tissue and help relax spasming muscles. Don't use deep work if your client is in a lot of pain.

It is also good to work in conjunction with another medical professional such as a medical doctor or chiropractor to address the client's issues. Working together usually creates a better result than working alone.

Dupuytren's Contracture (Trigger Finger)

Description

Dupuytren's contracture (also know as palmer fasciitis and trigger finger) is a connective tissue disorder that affects the palmer fascia of the hand. It usually mostly affects the long fibers of the palmar fascia that run parallel with the long tendons in the hand. The pathological process that starts this disorder is not known, but seems to start with an increase in fibroblasts that produce new collagen that form into nodules and fibrous restrictions.

In the early stages of the condition, fibrous nodules in the palmer region may be felt, the skin may pucker a bit in the area over the fibrous nodules, and the surface of the palm may be tender to palpation. There may be some limitation to extending the digits, either actively or passively.

In later stages of the condition, the flexion deformity will be clear and much more pronounced.

Myofascial trigger points in the palmaris longus or other forearm muscles can cause either pain or movement restrictions, which can make this condition worse.

Massage Considerations

Massage in the early stages of the condition is much more likely to help stop or slow down the development of this condition. Deep longitudinal stripping, myofascial work, and vigorous regular stretching are the most beneficial techniques. Also work with the forearm muscles and upper arm muscles that may also be contributing to tension in the palmer fascia may be beneficial.

If the condition is already severe, massage will not hurt, but it probably won't help much either.

Edema

Description

Edema is a local or systemic accumulation of interstitial fluid. It is associated with inflammation or poor circulation. It causes swelling and pain and is mostly found in legs and feet, but can be found in other areas of the body. The elevation of legs and rest seems to help with this condition.

Weak leg muscles can cause water retention, which makes older women particularly susceptible to this condition because leg muscles can deteriorate as a person ages. Varicose veins can also contribute to swelling.

Pitting edema is the most common form of edema. Edema is pitting when you press into a swollen area with a finger and the pressing causes an indentation that persists for a period of time after the pressure is released.

Non-pitting edema is less common. With this form of edema, pressure applied to the swollen area does not leave a persistent indentation.

Types of edema include:
- peripheral edema – this is the most common type. It occurs in the feet, ankles, and legs.
- pulmonary edema – an accumulation of fluid in the alveoli of the lungs.
- abdominal or peritoneal – an accumulation of fluid in the abdominal cavities.
- pleural effusion – an accumulation of fluid in the chest cavity.
- anasarca (extreme generalized edema) – general, widespread fluid in all tissues and cavities of the body at the same time.
- cerebral edema – an accumulation of excess fluid in the brain.

This condition is different from lymphedema, which is the result of damage to lymphatic structures and accumulation of proteins in the interstitial fluid.

Massage Considerations

Many types of edema contraindicate massage. Pitting edema is always a contraindication. There are types of massage that are designed to work with lymphatic flow (manual lymphatic drainage), but this is specialized work that you should study before doing.

Edema caused by the following conditions contraindicate massage:
- heart problems – the heart is overtaxed and not pumping blood at the proper volume.
- kidney problems – the kidneys are not filtering blood fast enough or completely enough due to chemical imbalance or mechanical obstruction.
- liver problems – the liver is congested due to chemical or mechanical issues.
- local infection – there is a risk of pushing pathogens into the lymphatic and circulatory systems before the body has had a chance to take care of it.
- blockage – mechanical blockage causing the edema. Could cause damage to delicate structures or break loose a blood clot or other debris. Types of blockage include:
  - edema associated with pregnancy
  - thrombus
  - embolism, deep vein thrombosis
  - lymph node damage

There are edemas that do benefit from massage work. Fluid retention due to a subacute musculoskeletal injury can benefit a great deal from massage. Also, a client confined to bed or partially immobilized for some reason can benefit from massage.

Manual lymphatic drainage (MLD) massage is a modality that is designed specifically for this type of body work.

You should be careful before starting work on these clients to make sure you understand what is really happening with the client and their type of edema before starting your massage.

Embolism/Thrombus

Description

Embolisms and thrombosis can be serious problems for clients. It is important that you are aware of these conditions and use extra caution when working with clients who have had either of these conditions recently.

An embolism is a traveling clot or collection of debris. It is formed in one part of the body and then moves to another part of the body where it can get stuck and cause a blockage.

A thrombosis is a lodged clot in a blood vessel and thrombophlebitis is an inflamed blood clot within a vein. Blood clots most often form in leg veins, but can start in other areas.

A pulmonary embolism occurs when an artery in a lung becomes blocked.

Emboli and thrombi that form on the arterial side of the systemic circuit are involved with cardiovascular disease. Having these can cause heart trouble and heart trouble can cause them.

Deep vein thrombosis (DVT) occurs when a blood clot forms in a deep vein (usually in the leg), which results in partially or complete blocked circulation. Symptoms include:
  • swelling

- pain
- discoloration
- abnormally hot skin at the affected area

However, almost half of DVT episodes have little if any symptoms.

Massage Considerations

When an embolism or thrombosis is present, avoid massage altogether. After the embolism or thrombosis is treated, gentle touch can be used with **caution**. Also be aware that if your client is taking an anticoagulant they may be more susceptible to bruising. Check with a doctor to make sure your client is cleared for massage.

Emphysema

Description

Emphysema is a condition in which the alveoli of the lungs become stretched out and inelastic. They merge with each other, decreasing the surface area of the lungs, destroying surrounding capillaries, and limited oxygen-carbon dioxide exchange. It is a part of chronic obstructive pulmonary disease (COPD).

Symptoms include:
- shortness of breath
- chronic dry coughing
- cyanosis (bluish, discoloration of the skin)
- susceptibility to respiratory infection

Massage Considerations

In the early stages, where skin is healthy and responsive and there are no heart problems or secondary infections, massage can be very beneficial.

In advanced cases, where a client has trouble breathing and shortness of breath, calming work can be beneficial. Clients may not be able to lay prone or supine. Stimulating strokes may not be advisable. The client may be more comfortable in a reclining chair, or other position. Find the best option for your client.

If a client has an inhaler, make sure it is close by and available during the massage.

Avoid any known triggers for asthma or allergies such as strong scents.

Fibromyalgia

Description

Fibromyalgia is a group of signs and symptoms that include chronic pain in muscles, tendons, ligaments, and other soft tissues causing widespread pain over the entire body. It is often seen in clients with other chronic diseases such as chronic fatigue syndrome, irritable bowel syndrome, migraine headaches, sleep disorders, and others. The incidence of this condition appears to increase with age.

Massage Considerations

Massage can be very beneficial for clients with fibromyalgia, but stay within the client's pain tolerance. Some clients will need an extremely light touch. Others will be able to handle deeper pressure. The pressure you use for your fibromyalgia clients depends on how they are feeling on a given day.

Do NOT use ice or perform ice massage. Any type of cold can exacerbate fibromyalgia symptoms.

Myofascial trigger points with tender areas might be better addressed with shorter, pulsing, gentler pressure instead of deep, aggressive pressure.

Circulatory massage with deep pressure can be helpful. Methods targeting pressure points can be very beneficial. Evaluate the tissue quality for resistance and check in with your client to determine the best approach for your client.

Gastroesophageal Reflux Disease (GERD)

Description

Gastroesophageal reflux disease (GERD) is caused when stomach contents rise into the esophagus. Occasional instances of this are not usually a problem, but frequent instances need to be evaluated by a doctor. This condition can cause or contribute to other problems including peptic ulcers, hiatal hernia, or possibly, esophageal cancer.

Massage Considerations

Massage can be helpful to clients with GERD, but caution must be used. When a client with this condition is on the massage table, gastric acid can splash back into the esophagus. You may need to adjust your massage session in one of the following ways:
- shorter, more frequent sessions
- working on the client at least two hours after a meal
- working in a massage chair
- propping your client up with a pillow when face up or face down

Your primary goal will be to make the client comfortable so he or she does not experience symptoms during the massage.

Work near the stomach should be conservative.

Guillain-Barre Syndrome

Description

Guillain-Barre syndrome involves the acute inflammation and destruction of the myelin layer of the peripheral nerves. It usually starts in the extremities and moves toward the trunk of the body. The onset of this condition is usually fast and severe with patients being fine, and then hospitalized within a few hours to a couple of days.

Massage Considerations

Avoid deep pressure because your client will be on blood thinners. Also remember that the client may be on pain medications, so they may not be able to properly measure the pressure they are receiving and if you are hurting them. Unless absolutely necessary, do not reposition the client.

Gout

Description

Gout is a type of inflammatory arthritis. It has a chemical cause rather than being caused by wear and tear or immune system problems. It results from the body being unable to handle the amount of uric acid being produced. There are three types of gout:

- metabolic gout – the kidneys are functioning properly, but there is too much uric acid for them to handle properly.
- renal gout – the uric acid load is normal, but the kidneys are not functioning properly.
- both – the kidneys are not functioning properly AND the amount of uric acid is too high.

Massage Considerations

Massage is contraindicated in the affected joint. Massage can do further damage to the joint and direct pressure can irritate and inflame the affected area. Massage elsewhere is beneficial.

Heart Attack

Description

A heart attack occurs when a portion of the cardiac muscle is damaged as a result of ischemia (decreased blood supply), which has starved and killed some of the muscle cells. The ischemia is usually a result of coronary artery disease or atherosclerosis of the coronary arteries.

Massage Considerations

Caution should be used, and how you work with the client will depend on the individual, how severe their heart attack was, and how your client is currently doing. If symptoms are still present, massage should be avoided. It is a good idea to get a doctor's clearance before beginning any massage work on someone who has had a recent heart attack.

Hypertension

Description

Hypertension is the technical term for high blood pressure. It is diagnosed when a person's blood pressure is consistently above 140 mm Hg systolic and/or 90 mm Hg diastolic. There are two types of hypertension:
- essential – not due to another pathology.
- secondary – a temporary complication from another condition.

Massage Considerations

If hypertension is not controlled, check with the client to see if he or she is cleared by their doctor for massage. If they are not, get the clearance before giving the massage. Once you have the clearance, choose modalities and plan your session to encourage relaxation. Trigger point and sports massage may cause an increase in blood pressure.

If the client has high blood pressure, but is NOT on medication, circulatory massage can be beneficial, especially if the client is physically active or encouraged to become physically active. You should make sure that kidney disease and other advanced cardiovascular problems are not the cause of the high blood pressure.

Comparing the type of body work you plan to do to your client's daily activities will help you determine what type of work to do in this situation.

Deep abdominal massage should be avoided so that you do not accidentally trip a vasovagal reaction. A vasovagal reaction is a reflex of the involuntary nervous system that causes the heart to slow down and blood pressure to drop, possibly causing your client to faint.

Hip Replacement

Description

The general term hip replacement is also known as total hip replacement, total hip joint replacement, hip replacement surgery, and total hip arthroplasty. It is a surgical procedure that removes a diseased hip joint and replaces it with an artificial joint. It is very common with mature adults.

Massage Considerations

It is good idea to get clearance from the client's physical therapist and/or doctor stating that massage is permitted or when to start massage sessions. Make sure your client is comfortable on the table during the session. Avoid any range of motion or stretches that affect the hip joint for about a year after the procedure to make sure the new hip is fully set in place.

Knee Replacement

Description

The general term knee replacement is also known as knee arthroplasty. It is a surgical procedure that replaces the weight-bearing surfaces of the knee joint. Your client can have a partial or full knee replacement. Knee replacements are common with mature adults.

Massage Considerations

It is a good idea to get clearance from the client's physical therapist and/or doctor that massage is permitted or when to start it. Make sure your client is comfortable on the table. A larger bolster may be helpful, especially when your client is prone. You can do some friction along the knee replacement scar to help remove scar tissue. Stretches and techniques to help the hamstrings relax are also helpful.

Techniques to help your client gain range of motion in knee joint are also helpful.

Osteoporosis

Description

Osteoporosis literally means porous bones, and is the weakening of the bones due to low bone mass and structural deterioration of bone tissue. This condition exists when calcium is pulled out of the bones faster than it is replaced and the calcium deposits in the bone tissue become dangerously thin.

Depending on the location and amount of osteoporosis, the client may be in pain from muscular stress.

More women than men get this condition.

Massage Considerations

Moderation of your pressure will be key when working with a client with osteoporosis. Lighter pressure is very important, especially if the osteoporosis is extensive. Make sure you understand where the osteoporosis is located and

that you communicate with your client to make sure you are not hurting them.

Parkinson Disease

NOTE: This condition is more commonly found when doing geriatric massage. However, you may run into mature adults

---

who are in the early stages of this disorder. In the early stages, the type of massage you perform probably won't be much different from a regular massage. In the later stages, though, your massage can be vastly different.

Description

Parkinson disease (PD) is a movement disorder that affects about one percent of people over 60. It affects men more often than women. It is a neurological movement disorder that affects the substantia nigra (small area in the basil ganglia in the brain), the key to the coordination of muscle movements. The nerve tissue degenerates creating a reduction in neurotransmitter production in the CNS.

Tremors are a common sign of PD, but the disorder also causes stiffness or slowing of movement.

Early on, symptoms of the disease include shaking, rigidity, slow movement, and difficulty walking. As the disease progresses, thinking and behavioral problems may occur. Dementia and depression often occur in the advanced stages of the disease.

Massage Considerations

Massage is generally supported and good for the PD client. You should work within the client's tolerance levels both for pressure and flexibility. Keep in mind that your client's range of motion and movements may not be as good as other clients and you may have to adjust how you massage certain areas.

Massage may affect the need for some kinds of medication, so it is important to check with the client's primary care physician or caregiver to understand what medications your client is taking and, if necessary, plan your sessions according to their recommendations

Peripheral Neuropathy

Description

Peripheral neuropathy (PN) is a symptom or complication of another condition. It often starts with numbness and tingling bilaterally in the toes and feet and then progresses to the lower legs. Fingers and hands might be next and then the arms. It usually affects the longest nerves first and shorter nerves later.

There are many causes for this condition, but not all causes are known. Chemotherapy and diabetes are known to be causes of peripheral neuropathy. It can also be caused by injury, infection, systemic disease, and toxic exposure.

Massage Considerations

This is a tricky area for massage therapists. Usually, the client has reduced or no feeling in their extremities so they cannot give you proper feedback on pressure. However, if you have a light enough touch, you may still be able to massage your client very gently in the areas affected by the PN. This will help increase circulation in the affected areas and your client may enjoy any remaining sensations.

You MUST use extreme caution and make sure any work you do does not harm the client. Judge each client on their own individual issues.

Post-Polio Syndrome

Description

Post-polio syndrome (PPS) affect polio survivors many years after they have recovered from an initial case of polio. It causes weakening in the muscles that were originally affected by the first occurrence of polio, but also attacks muscles that did not appear to be affected in the first case. It is not contagious.

Because polio has been eradicated from the US, this condition should also eventually disappear.

Massage Considerations

There is no numbness associated with PPS so there are no concerns on sensory input for performing massage. PPS clients may have changed their walking and moving habits to take advantage of their stronger muscles, so massage can help relieve tension and soreness from newly or differently used muscles as well as help nourish and refresh muscles weakened due to the condition.

Postural Deviations

Description

Postural deviations are overdeveloped thoracic or lumbar curve or a lateral curve in the spine. These conditions include:

- hyperkyphosis (humpback, Dowager's hump) – overdeveloped thoracic curve
- hyperlordosis (swayback) – over-pronounced lumbar curve
- scoliosis – S, C, or reverse-C curve in the spine

These conditions can result from either a functional or a structural problem. Many times, functional and structural deviations are caused by tightness in the soft tissue that pulls the spine out of alignment. Functional deviations can also be caused by structural deviations in other parts of the body. Usually, these conditions can be corrected when caught early.

Massage Considerations

Massage is very helpful in relieving the pain and stress of muscles affected by these conditions. If massage is used early enough in the development of these conditions, it might be possible to help reverse the problem with massage. However, the longer the condition continues, the harder it will be to undo the damage and at some point, your primary goal will just be to make the client feel better.

Stroke

NOTE: This condition is more of a geriatric massage condition, but can happen at any time, changing your mature adult massage client into a geriatric massage client.

Description

Stroke is also known as a cerebrovascular accident (CVA) and is an interruption of blood flow to a specific part of the brain. There are two types of stroke: brain hemorrhage and brain ischemia. Brain ischemia is the most common type of stroke and has four main causes:

- atherostenosis is the narrowing in the major arteries feeding the brain, which causes a decrease in blood flow
- occlusion of small penetrating arteries deep within the brain
- embolism
- hypoperfusion or hypotensive shock is caused by poor cardiac output or general system failure

Transient ischemic attack (TIA) refers to mini-strokes. They are considered precursors or warning signs for a future stroke.

Massage Considerations

You will want to work with your client's health care team to make sure your client is cleared for massage. You probably won't be able to do more than a 30-minute massage, especially if the stroke is fairly recent. Depending on how your client recovers, longer massages may be possible later on in his or her recovery.

Massage will not cause a stroke, but you need to apply caution. Make sure you have an accurate medical history, including current medications. If there is a chance of blood clots, extreme caution should be used and it may contraindicate massage. If your client is on a blood thinner, light strokes should be used and deep tissue or heavy pressure should be avoided to avoid bruising or hurting your client.

Training in this type of geriatric massage is recommended.

Varicose Veins

Description

Varicose veins are distended, twisty, or ropy superficial veins. Blood collects in the veins when valves that support blood flow against gravity are damaged. This blood collection causes the vein to be stretched, distorted, and weakened.

Spider veins are similar to varicose veins, but they are smaller veins and closer to the skin's surface.

Sometimes the symptoms of varicose veins are only cosmetic, but some people will have pain, aching, and fatigue in the legs, particularly when walking. Calf muscles may cramp especially at night. Blood clots are more likely to develop in varicose veins.

Massage Considerations

If there is broken skin, ulceration, or phlebitis, do not work directly on the varicose veins. If there is ulceration, lymphatic drainage and circulatory work can be used proximal to the lesion. Myofascial release techniques can be used at the margin of venous ulceration to help soften and release areas of hardening, which can lead to the freer movement of skin and underlying tissue.

In general, avoid deep pressure, especially if the varicose veins are particularly serious. Gentler circulatory work can be beneficial.

Chapter 7 – Working with Hospice Clients

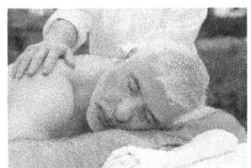 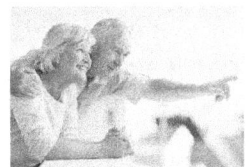 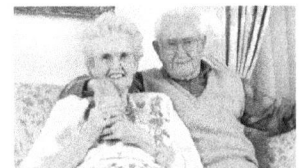

Hospice clients fall more into the category of geriatric massage, but you may run into clients in hospice care the more you work with mature adults. Whether they are in hospice care in their homes, in a hospice facility, or in a nursing home or hospital, they are under the hospice umbrella because they are not expected to live much longer.

In this stage, the goal is to make the patient/client as comfortable as possible during their last weeks and days.

Some people may have trouble working with these clients. It can be hard to be with a person you know is dying. However, it can also be one of the most rewarding ways to do massage because you help make these clients' last days better with your touch.

I've only worked with a couple of hospice clients, but my experiences seem to be reflected in stories I've heard from other massage therapists who work with those in hospice. The massage therapist is a bright spot in the client's day. At this point in their life, the client usually isn't able to get around and are pretty much bedbound. A lot of the touch and attention these people get is more about helping them move or turn over, cleaning them, medical monitoring, and poking and prodding. Family members may not know how to deal with them and they may be afraid to touch or hug them. Many hospice clients can use good, caring touch and a reminder that they are a human being who deserves care and attention.

I truly enjoyed the time I spent with my clients in hospice care. They were both wonderful ladies whom I would have liked to have gotten to know better. Even though it was sad when they passed, I am happy to know that they are no longer suffering and are in a better place.

Primary Concerns

Your primary concern when working with clients in hospice care is making them feel better. At this point you're not trying to fix anything, you are just giving your client a soothing massage.

You want to be aware of any contraindications that might prevent you from massaging your client altogether or only in a certain area. Although your client is in the last stages of life, you certainly don't want to make their condition worse.

Your massage sessions will most likely be modified with regard to where you do the massage and how long the session lasts. While I have done table massage with hospice clients, most of the time you will probably end up working with your client in their bed or in a hospital bed.

You will also adjust your massage to the physical and energy levels of your client. Especially as the client gets closer to the end of life, you may only do 20 or 30 minutes (or even less) of massage and you may only work small areas like hands, feet, and neck, but your client will love it!

Doctor's Approval

Many doctors know and understand the power of massage, but you may still run into some resistance from a doctor when you try to do massage with their patient who is under hospice care. Honest and open communication can really help in this instance.

One of the therapists I had in one of my CE classes told me her story of how she worked with a doctor. She had been working with a client for quite a while and the client really looked forward to her massages. Her doctor, though, was against his patient receiving a massage! Instead of getting angry and huffy with the doctor, this therapist approached the doctor and said, "Can you help me understand? I want to learn."

The therapist explained, "I was just going to do a little rubbing on her feet, would that cause a problem?" The doctor thought about it and said, "No, that should be okay." Then she said, "Well, what about the hands?" And the doctor thought again, and again, said, "That should be okay." In the end, the therapist was able to give her client the massage the client wanted, but she also got the buy-in from the doctor.

What I take away from this story is that both the massage therapist and the doctor wanted to help their client/patient. The doctor probably didn't know what the therapist had in mind at first and didn't want to see his patient harmed. The massage therapist also didn't want to harm her client, and she was pretty sure she wouldn't, but she showed the doctor that she was willing to learn something she didn't know. In the end, I think both parties felt good about what had happened and the client won!

Pay

A lot of Hospice work will be on a volunteer basis. However, if the client's family brings you in to do a massage, that will most likely be paid work. If you want to do hospice massage on a volunteer basis, it is a great calling and can be very fulfilling work. On the other hand, there is also nothing wrong with being paid for working with clients in hospice care. However you do it, know that you will be a positive and bright spot in the day of someone who is preparing for the end of their life.

Chapter 8 – The Death of a Client

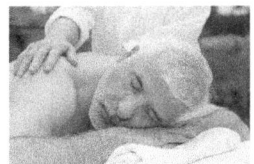 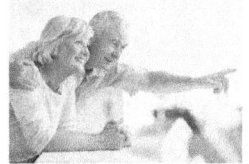 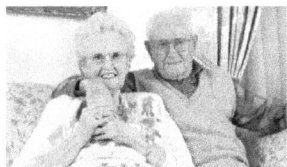

Although anyone can die at any time, the chances of it happening when we are younger are fairly low. When you are working with mature adults, though, you have a higher chance of having clients who will pass away. Although many mature adults are healthy and active, they are older and more susceptible to severe health problems.

Massage is an intimate service and when you have clients you have seen for a long time, having one of them die can be difficult to handle. You will probably know a lot about your client like how they grew up, what they did with their life, who their children and grandchildren are. Even in a professional relationship, you will grow attached to your clients.

The important thing to understand is that you will have to deal with the death of a client at some point and you will have to find a way to deal with it that works for you.

The first thing that you have to accept is that it is going to happen. Not every week or every month, but you may lose one or two of your clients a year (maybe more if most of your clients are closer to the geriatric stage). But, if most of your clients are on the younger side and still in good health, it is less likely that you will have many clients every year who pass away.

The second thing you will have to figure out is how to deal with the death of a client. For some of your clients, this may not be as hard. If you haven't worked with them for an extended period, you probably won't be as attached—not that you won't feel the loss, but if you've only been seeing them for a few months, there may not be as much of an emotional attachment. Or, if your client is very old and has had a full life, you can take a philosophical approach knowing that client had a long, fulfilled life and can now rest. Many of my clients who have passed away have fallen into one of these two categories.

However, I now have clients that I've been seeing for over four years and expect to continue seeing for a long time. I love almost all my clients and I know about their lives and I know a lot of their children and even some of their grandchildren. I know that for these core clients, when they pass (which I hope won't be for a long, long, LONG time) I will be very upset and it will be very hard for me. It will be like losing a friend or member of my own family. And because most of my clients are so healthy and active, I can't even imagine one of them passing away any time soon. I just don't think of them as old, even if they are in their 70s and 80s!

The important thing to remember is that this is not a regular occurrence when working with mature adults, but it does happen more often than when working with younger clients. I wanted to include this topic in this book so you would have a complete idea of what working with mature adults can be like and be prepared. Most of your mature adult clients will be with you for a long time and your massages will help them live as long as possible. Enjoy your time with them!

Chapter 8 – The Death of a Client

Chapter 9 – Marketing to Mature Adults

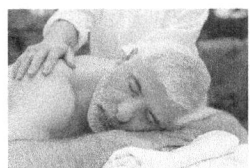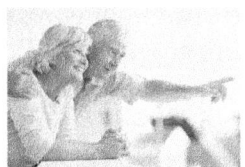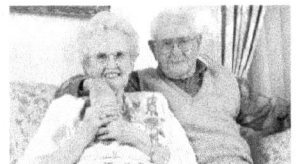

As with any other group you target in your business, you will need to figure out how to gain new mature adult clients. What works for one target market group, may not work for another. This chapter includes some marketing ideas for mature adults and how well they've worked for me. Many of them may work for you, and, of course, you may find other ways that work for you that I haven't even thought of!

Fairs

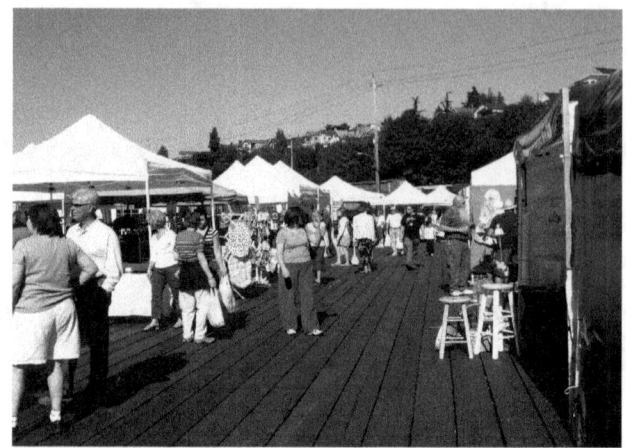

Outdoor Fair

This is one of my favorite and best ways to get new clients. Vendor, health, and community fairs allow you to meet a lot of potential clients in one place. These events are fun and the people who attend are interested in looking at the booths and tables of the vendors who are there. Not everyone will be interested in what you have to offer, but if the fair is targeted specifically to mature adults, you will have a greater chance of building your client base.

At these events, you can offer chair massage, but if you do, I would recommend that you have another person who can also man your booth and talk to people who are walking by while you are massaging. It is very hard to market and do chair massage at the same time! I usually just focus on my marketing. I talk to the people who are interested and tell them about what I have to offer and my rates. When potential clients mention a specific problem, I can tell them if I think I will be able to help and how I would help them. This engages the client and they will be more likely to book an appointment.

Having a special rate for fair participants is a WONDERFUL way to entice potential clients to try you out. I recommend a half-priced massage (I rarely give free massages!). Make sure you put a time limit on the special rate and make it clear that it is for new clients only. While you will have some clients who just want their half-priced massage and will never call you again, you will gain several clients who will become regular clients after trying you out!

You will have to find the right event for this type of marketing to succeed. I've been to some fairs that haven't brought me in any new clients. I attend every vendor fair and health fair at the Sun City community I work in, though, and those are always well worth the time and money I spend on them.

This marketing method has been the best and most successful way I've used to grow my business. When you attend the right fair event it will be one of the most efficient ways to get new clients!

Referrals

There are two different types of referrals: those from your clients and those from other businesses. Both referral types are wonderful because you are being recommended by people that your potential client trusts.

Certainly your clients know what you have done for them and they want to spread the word about you. When they tell their friends, their friends will want to try you. When you offer a reward for your client spreading the word (such as $10.00 of their next massage for every referral who gets a massage from you), they will want to spread the word even more!

If you can get other businesses, especially ones related to what you do, such as chiropractors and physical therapists, to refer clients to you, this is another great way to grow your client list. If a potential client really likes the professional who is referring to you, they will seriously consider calling you. Of course, you will want to reciprocate with these other professionals, so make sure you believe the people you are referring to are people you would go to yourself (if you don't already go to them).

As with most marketing techniques, this type can take a little while to grow. It may seem slow at first, but as you get more clients, more people will spread the word about you. This will then, hopefully, put you in the enviable position of having more clients than you know what to do with!

A great thing about this type of marketing is that, except for rewarding your clients who refer to you, you don't have to spend a lot of money (and the more referral bonuses you pay out, the more clients you will have and the more money you will make).

Classified Ads

When I bought the client list to get my business started, the therapist I bought the list from also shared with me how she had grown her business in the community she worked in (where I would be taking over). One of the things she told me was that she kept a classified ad in the monthly magazine that went to every house in the community.

At first, I was surprised. I didn't think anyone really looked at classified ads any more. But what I found out was that in this retirement community, that magazine was a regularly-used resource for that community's residents, and yes, that included the classified ads section! Every house I go into in this community, I usually see this magazine on a table somewhere in the house and my clients have told me they look at it every time it comes out and use it for reference to locate businesses.

There are some months I don't get any calls from my ad, but other months I get several calls. It has been one of the best ways to advertise my business. It also keeps my name in the community and, if a client can't find my business card, they know they can look in that magazine to get my phone number.

This method has worked well for me and I usually make my money back on it with new clients. I don't know if this will change in the future as more mature adults move to online resources, but for now it's a great marketing tool!

Networking with Others in the Senior Industry

The more people who know what you do, the more clients you will have! If you can find a networking group that focuses on the senior industry (those who cater to mature adults), this will help you a great deal. I joined a group that included businesses such as real estate agents, insurance agents, 55-and-older communities, home health agencies, independent living and assisted living communities, and many other businesses, all of whom catered to mature adults. This was great because we were all targeting the same market, but we had different skills and offerings for mature adults. I learned about different options I could mention to my clients should they ask and the other businesses learned about what I did to pass on to their customers and clients.

This type of marketing doesn't give you immediate clients, but if you network regularly, you will find that your name will get around and you will be able to help others who will help you!

Direct Marketing

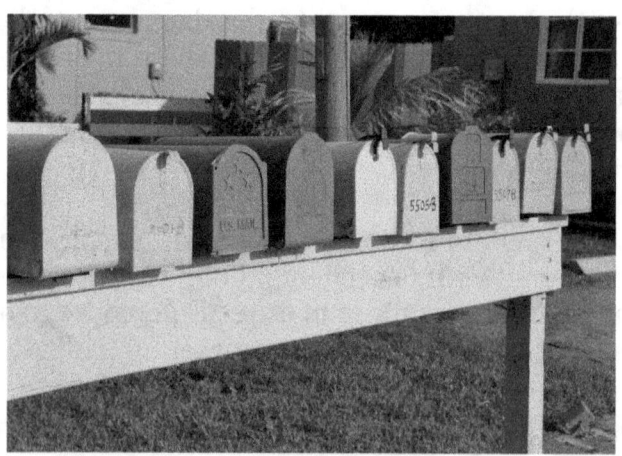

A Postcard in Every Mailbox!

Direct mail, such as postcards or other types of mailings, isn't always successful these days. However, with older adults it can still have an impact. As with most types of marketing, though, you will need to be persistent with it. One postcard mailing probably won't bring you in many (if any) calls. It may take three or four (or more) mailings.

I personally haven't had a lot of luck with this method, but it might work for you. Just remember that this type of marketing comes with a fairly high cost. You will have to print up the postcards or mailers and then you have postage and, as stated above, you will probably have to do several mailings. For a small community, it might be worth trying, but a larger community will cost you a LOT of money.

Internet (Future)

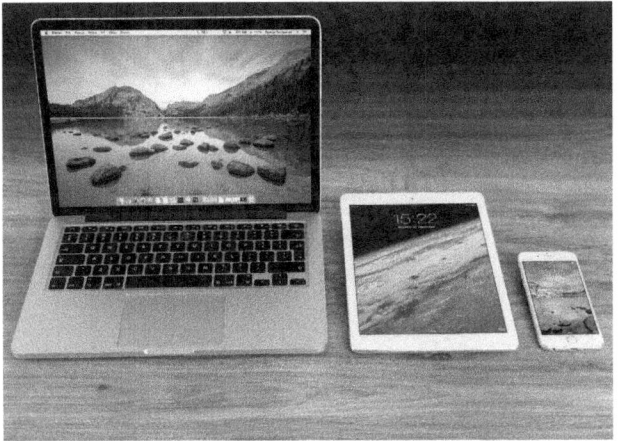

Online is the Future

Although some older adults are online and are enjoying the Internet, many still mostly use email and Facebook only to keep in touch with family, if they're online at all. They are not major surfers and they don't look to the Internet to find new businesses. So, today, Internet marketing is not as effective if you are targeting mature adults. If you target the children of older adults, however, you might have more success.

In the next five to ten years, though, the Internet will become a bigger player in marketing to the mature adult. The baby boomers are much more tech savvy than their predecessors. I expect by 2020 you will need to have a larger Internet and social media (or whatever is big then!) presence to market to mature adults.

It's a good idea to get your online presence set up today. If you are new to websites and using social media for your business, this is the time to learn. That way you will be ready when it is really important!

Chapter 10 – Final Thoughts

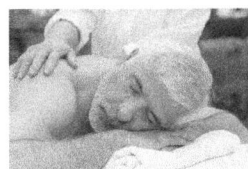 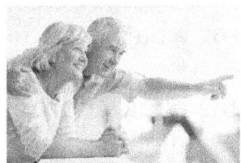 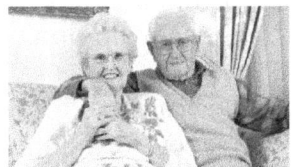

Massaging mature adults is a great way to practice massage. You will never find a more grateful group of people to work with. Not only will you be able to improve the lives of some wonderful people, you will get to know some fascinating individuals as well.

You will find that many people who are over 60 are still in excellent health and use massage as a way to keep themselves healthy. For more frail clients or clients with health issues, massage can make a big difference in the quality of their lives. Whether it's a relaxation massage or therapeutic session, or a little of both, you will have clients who love and appreciate what you do for them.

Treating each client as an individual and keeping the 4 Cs in mind when working with your clients will serve you well when working with mature adults. Never judge a mature adult by their age or their gray hair or wrinkles.

The mature adult population is growing and will continue to grow through 2030. The opportunity is there for you to have a thriving business working with this group of people. Knowing how to work with this population (what you learned in this book) will give you a competitive edge against other therapists who don't know what you now know.

I hope you have found this book informative and helpful. Thank you for taking the time to read it and good luck working with your own mature adults!

Bibliography

Chapter 3

1. JoEllen M. Sefton, PhD, A. T. C., C.M.T., Ceren Yarar, PhD, P.T., and Jack W. Berry, PhD, "Six Weeks of Massage Therapy Produces Changes in Balance, Neurological and Cardiovascular Measures in Older Persons," *International Journal of Therapeutic Massage and Bodywork* c.5(3) (2012), accessed January 11, 2016, PMC:PMC3457720.

Chapter 6

1. Ruth Werner, *A Massage Therapist's Guide to Pathology*, Fourth Edition (Baltimore: Lippincott Williams & Wilkins, 2009)
2. "The Power of Touch for ALS," AMTA, accessed January 11, 2016, https://www.amtamassage.org/articles/1/News/detail/3001
3. "Massage and Lou Gehrig's Disease," Pacific College of Oriental Medicine, accessed January 11, 2016, http://www.pacificcollege.edu/news/blog/2014/12/06/massage-and-lou-gehrigs-disease
4. "Educating Yourself: Massaging a Client with ALS," Massage Today, accessed January 11, 2016, http://www.massagetoday.com/mpacms/mt/article.php?id=14889
5. "Bursitis," University of Maryland Medical Center, accessed January 11, 2016, http://umm.edu/health/medical/altmed/condition/bursitis

6. "Massage Therapy for Bursitis," Massage Education Guide, accessed January 11, 2016, http://www.massage-education.com/bursitis.html

7. "Crohn's Disease Treatment," Everyday Healh, accessed January 11, 2016, http://www.everydayhealth.com/crohns-disease/treatment/

8. "What You Should Know About Decubitus Ulcers," Healthline, accessed January 11, 2016, http://www.healthline.com/health/pressure-ulcer#Causes3

9. "Massage Therapy for Breast Cancer Patients," Pacific College of Oriental Medicine, accessed January 11, 2016, http://www.pacificcollege.edu/news/blog/2014/11/06/massage-therapy-breast-cancer-patients#sthash.5u44snFl.dpuf

10. "Faqs: Can massage spread cancer?," Tracy Walton & Associates, accessed January 11, 2016, http://www.tracywalton.com/faqs-new/

11. "Massage," breastcancer.org, accessed January 11, 2016, http://www.breastcancer.org/treatment/comp_med/types/massage

12. "Oncology: Bodywork for Cancer Patients," massagetherapy.com, accessed January 11, 2016, http://www.massagetherapy.com/articles/index.php/article_id/960/Oncology%3A-Bodywork-for-Cancer-Patients

13. "Treating Depression with Massage," Massage Today, accessed January 11, 2016, http://www.massagetoday.com/mpacms/mt/article.php?id=13933

14. "Diabetes: Massage as an Adjunct Treatment," massagetherapy.com, accessed January 11, 2016, http://www.massagetherapy.com/articles/index.php/article_id/96/Diabetes

15. "Degenerative Spine: Massage Therapy," Laser Spine Institute®, accessed January 11, 2016, https://www.laserspineinstitute.com/articles/degenerative_spine/massage/459/

16. "Degenerative Disc Disease Massage," massagetherapyreference.com, accessed January 11, 2016, http://www.massagetherapyreference.com/degenerative-disc-disease-massage/

17. "Dupuytren's Contracture," Massage Today, accessed January 11, 2016, http://www.massagetoday.com/mpacms/mt/article.php?id=14648

18. "Edema and how Massage Therapy may help!," massage-education.com, accessed January 11, 2016, http://www.massage-education.com/edema.html

19. "Pulmonary Embolism Discharge Information," Summit Medical Group, accessed January 11, 2016, http://www.summitmedicalgroup.com/library/adult_care/ac-pulmonaryembolism_dc/

20. "Emphysema," The Massage Source, accessed January 11, 2016, http://www.themassagesource.com/health-concerns/emphysema

21. "The Subtleties of Breath-ing," massagetherapy.com, accessed January 11, 2016, http://www.massagetherapy.com/articles/index.php/article_id/1368/The-Subtleties-of-Breath-ing

22. "Respiratory Diseases," Massage Pathology Chronicles, accessed January 11, 2016, http://massage-pathology-chronicles.com/2009/11/13/respiratory-diseases/

23. "Treating Fibromyalgia," massagetherapy.com, accessed January 11, 2016, http://www.massagetherapy.com/articles/index.php/article_id/644/Treating-Fibromyalgia

24. "Massage Therapy and Fibromyalgia," Pacific College of Oriental Medicine, accessed January 11, 2016, http://www.pacificcollege.edu/news/press-releases/2015/05/05/massage-therapy-and-fibromyalgia

25. "Fibromyalgia Part 2: Nine Massage Techniques," Institute for Integrative Healthcare, accessed January 11, 2016, http://www.integrativehealthcare.org/mt/archives/2006/01/nine_massage_te.html

26. "How Massage Can Relieve Heartburn Symptoms," Institute for Integrative Healthcare, accessed January 11, 2016, http://www.integrativehealthcare.org/mt/archives/2007/08/how_massage_imp.html

27. "Guillain-Barre Syndrome: Is there a role for massage therapy? Part 2," Massage Therapy Canada, accessed January 11, 2016, http://www.massagetherapycanada.com/technique/guillain-barre-syndrome-1802

28. "Gout and Massage," Gout and You, accessed January 11, 2016, http://goutandyou.com/gout-and-massage/

29. "Why Massages Really Do Keep You Healthy: A Cardiologist Explains," mindbodygreen, accessed January 11, 2016, http://www.mindbodygreen.com/0-11315/why-massages-really-do-keep-you-healthy-a-cardiologist-explains.html

30. "The Benefits of Massage for Hypertension," Pacific College of Oriental Medicine, accessed January 11, 2016, http://www.pacificcollege.edu/news/blog/2015/01/24/benefits-massage-hypertension

31. "The Ups and Downs of Blood Pressure: Effects of Varying Types of Massage Therapy," massagetherapy.com, accessed January 11, 2016, http://www.massagetherapy.com/articles/index.php/article_id/1267/The-Ups-and-Downs-of-Blood-Pressure%3A-Effects-of-Varying-Types-of-Massage-Therapy

32. "Massage + Anterior Hip Replacement," amtamassage.org, accessed January 11, 2016, https://www.amtamassage.org/articles/3/MTJ/detail/3057

33. "Benefits of Massage," Arthritis Foundation[SM], accessed January 11, 2016, http://www.arthritis.org/living-with-arthritis/treatments/natural/other-therapies/massage/massage-benefits.php

34. "Remedies for Osteoarthritis," amtamassage.org, accessed January 11, 2016, https://www.amtamassage.org/articles/3/MTJ/detail/1768

35. "Massage for Osteoarthritis," Pacific College of Oriental Medicine, accessed January 11, 2016, http://www.pacificcollege.edu/news/blog/2015/01/31/massage-osteoarthritis

36. "Doubling Bodywork's Effectiveness Against Osteoporosis," Institute for Integrative Healthcare, accessed January 11, 2016, http://www.integrativehealthcare.org/mt/archives/2011/06/doubling_bodywo.html

37. "Osteoporosis and Hyperkyphosis: What Does Calcium Have to Do With it?," massagetherapy.com, accessed January 11, 2016, http://www.massagetherapy.com/articles/index.php/article_id/1260/Osteoporosis-and-Hyperkyphosis%3A-What-Does-Calcium-Have-to-Do-With-It

38. "A Strong Combination," massagetherapy.com, accessed January 11, 2016, http://www.massagetherapy.com/articles/index.php/article_id/289/Bodywork-and-Parkinson%92s-Patients

39. "Peripheral Neuropathy; A Panoply of Problems," abmp.com, accessed January 11, 2016, https://www.abmp.com/textonlymags/article.php?article=681

40. "A Massage Protocol for Peripheral Neuropathy," Massage Today, accessed January 11, 2016, http://www.massagetoday.com/mpacms/mt/article.php?id=14537

41. "Skin Cancer: Practitioners as Lookouts," massagetherapy.com, accessed January 11, 2016, http://www.massagetherapy.com/articles/index.php/article_id/1025/Skin-Cancer%3A-Practitioners-as-Lookouts

42. "Massage Therapists and the Detection of Skin Cancer in Clients," Massage Today, accessed January 11, 2016, http://www.massagetoday.com/mpacms/mt/article.php?id=14711

43. "Massage After Stroke," Stroke-Rehab.com, accessed January 11, 2016, http://www.stroke-rehab.com/massage-after-stroke1.html

44. "Stroke Rehab, Part 2: Coming Back," massagetherapy.com, accessed January 11, 2016, http://www.massagetherapy.com/articles/index.php/article_id/298/Stroke-Rehab-Part-2

45. "What about Varicose Veins?," Massage Today, accessed January 11, 2016, http://www.massagetoday.com/mpacms/mt/article.php?id=10245

46. "Hip Replacement," PhysioAdvisor.com, accessed January 11, 2016, http://www.physioadvisor.com.au/14124650/hip-replacement-total-hip-replacement-physioad.htm

47. "Knee Replacement," PhysioWorks.com, accessed January 11, 2016, http://physioworks.com.au/injuries-conditions-1/knee-replacement-knee-arthroplasty

48. "How is Rheumatoid Arthritis Treated?," National Institute of Arthritis and Musculoskeletal and Skin Diseases, accessed January 11, 2016, http://www.niams.nih.gov/Health_Info/Rheumatic_Disease/default.asp#ra_10

49. "What is Edema," MedicineNet.com, accessed January 11, 2016, http://www.medicinenet.com/edema/article.htm#what_is_edema

50. "embolism," The Free Dictionary, accessed January 11, 2016, http://medical-dictionary.thefreedictionary.com/embolism

51. "Hypertension: Massage Indication or Contraindication," Institute for Integrative Healthcare, accessed January 11, 2016, http://www.integrativehealthcare.org/mt/archives/2007/01/hypertension_ma.html

52. "Definition of Vasovagal Reaction," MedicineNet.com, accessed January 11, 2016, http://www.medicinenet.com/script/main/art.asp?articlekey=7713

53. "Post-Polio Syndrome Fact Sheet," National Institute of Neurological Disorders and Strok, accessed January 11, 2016, http://www.ninds.nih.gov/disorders/post_polio/detail_post_polio.htm

Continue the Education Journey

For more information on this and other topics and to earn CE credits, check out Mary Duval's website, www.maryduval.com.

This site provides information about Mary's upcoming in-person CE classes, online CE courses, and upcoming continuing education topics.

You can follow Mary Duval on Facebook at: https://www.facebook.com/Mary-Duval-InstructorCE-Provider-418642331646791/.

Bibliography